ESSENTIAL MACROBIOTICS

THE UNIVERSAL WAY OF SELF-REALIZATION

DON MATESZ
with
TRACY MATESZ

ESSENTIAL MACROBIOTICS

The Universal Way of Self-Realization

Don Matesz, M.A., M.S., L.Ac.
with some text by
Tracy Matesz, M.S., L.Ac.

INTEGRITY PRESS
2016

ESSENTIAL MACROBIOTICS

First Edition

Copyright © 2016 Donald A. Matesz

All rights reserved

ISBN-13: 978-1535363372

ISBN-10: 1535363371

No part of this book may be reproduced or transmitted in any form or by any means, electronic or mechanical, including photocopying, recording, or by any information storage and retrieval system, except for brief excerpts for the purposes of review and commentary, without written permission from the copyright holder.

Cover Image Copyright: halimqd/Shutterstock

Authorship Note

Don Matesz composed the text of chapters 1-4 and 7-9 and did all the layout and design of the entire book. Tracy Minton Matesz helped with editing and design of the entire book and contributed some of the text in chapters 5 and 6.

Contents

Notice ii

Preface iii

Introduction 1

1: Macrobiotic Mindset 10

2: Natural Law 27

3: Health & Sickness 46

4: Macrobiotic Diet 56

5: Basic Menus 87

6: Basic Recipes 92

7: Harmonizing Yin and Yang 105

8: Macrobiotic Fitness 110

9: Macrobiotic Lifestyle 120

Bibliography 136

NOTICE

Diet has a powerful effect on health and fitness. If you are seriously ill or on medications, consult a health care provider knowledgable about nutrition and its health effects and about your medications before you make any changes to your diet or exercise program. You remain always responsible for your choices, actions, and their consequences. This book serves as educational information only and does not substitute for the guidance of a health care professional familiar with your unique situation. Nothing herein is to be construed as a diagnosis or treatment plan for any individual's unique physical condition.

PREFACE

Most likely you come to this book with a load of beliefs about reality, religion, science, politics, government, nature, and yourself. Have you ever taken an inventory of them? Do you know how many you acquired before you had enough experience or knowledge to properly evaluate them? How many do you believe simply because you heard others repeat the belief innumerable times, or because you needed to accept and regurgitate the belief in order to "pass" a test or grade or get a "degree"? How many did you accept because it was required of you to do so in order to remain accepted and supported by your family or tribe? How many are unjustified traditions or dogmas from scriptures (which may include science textbooks) written by men with ulterior motives? How many of your beliefs actually correspond to Reality, and how many project illusions?

Whether they are true or not, your beliefs motivate your actions and shape your experience. If your beliefs and actions are not aligned with Reality, you're like a sailor whose boat sails are not aligned with the wind. If you aren't getting what you want out of life, its time to ditch the beliefs that prevent you from prospering.

But I don't want you to "believe" anything I have written in this book. This is not a book of beliefs. It is a book about aligning with Reality, principles of Natural Law and practices based on the Truth. You probably wonder how I define Truth. Very simply: Truth is that which no one can deny or doubt because it is or aligns with Reality.

Some readers, particularly those highly educated in the modern sciences, will likely be tempted to immediately reject some of the ideas presented herein because they will conflict with the conventionally approved scientific world view. If you find yourself in a knee-jerk rejection of anything in this book, I invite you to suspend your reaction long enough to entertain and evaluate the ideas in relation to Reality and patterns of phenomena.

Avoid comparing the ideas in this book only to the theories you were taught by "authorities" and forced to accept in order to get good grades and advance in the tightly controlled educational system. Instead, compare them to Reality using logic, introspection, and direct experience. Try to refute the principles set forth by reference to Reality, not theory or doctrine. To paraphrase a Buddhist sutta: If you see and know that any idea is refuted by Reality, harmful to Self and others, and rejected by healthy, happy, benevolent, and wise people, drop it.[1] Rather than believing, adhere to Truth and Virtue as only these will set you free.

---

[1] The Kalama Sutta; Anguttara Nikaya, Tika Nipata, Mahavagga, Sutta No. 65.
<http://www.accesstoinsight.org/lib/authors/soma/wheel008.html>

The highest good is like water.
Water gives life to the ten thousand things and does not strive.
It flows in places men reject and so resembles the Tao.
In dwelling, stay close to the land.
In meditation, go deep in the heart.
In dealing with others, be gentle and kind.
In speech, be true.
In ruling, be just.
In daily life, be competent.
In action, be aware of the time and the season.

No fight: No blame.

TAO TE CHING
Chapter 8

INTRODUCTION
The Degeneration of Humanity and Nature

Modern man has produced an advanced technological society with many wondrous luxuries. We can fly hundreds of miles in an hour, explore the depths of the ocean, and transmit audio and visual messages across the world in moments. We produce more food than ever, and we live in regions previously uninhabitable due to advanced indoor climate control. We seem to be on top of the world.

If you consider only these apparent successes, it seems logical to conclude that this technological advancement and the modern world view that produced it have been proven correct. However, a deeper investigation reveals that this apparent progress has been accompanied by physical, mental and moral degeneration of humanity and degradation of the life-support systems of the Earth.

Rates of sexually transmitted diseases reached an unprecedented high in the U.S. in 2015.[1] About 20 million new STD infections occur every year in the U.S., half of these in young adults aged 15-24, and the organisms present in these diseases have become drug resistant.[2] These diseases can cause blindness, infertility, stillbirths, and birth defects.

In the U.S., birth defects affect 3% of babies and are the leading cause of infant death, accounting for 20% of all infant deaths.[3] Dental defects, malocclusions, and decay are nearly universal.[4] About 20% of the population suffers from digestive diseases.[5] About 9% of the U.S. population has diabetes.[6] One-third of all U.S. deaths in 2013 were caused by heart disease, stroke, or other cardiovascular diseases.[7] In 2016, there will be about 4,620 new cases of cancer diagnosed, and 1,630 deaths from cancer every day in the U.S..[8] The leading cancer sites are prostate, breast, lung, colorectal, uterus, and urinary bladder. About 3% of the U.S. population has an autoimmune disorder.[9]

Eight percent of U.S. children engage in non-suicidal self-injury.[10] Major depression affected 7% of all U.S. adults in 2015.[11] Between 1999 and 2014, the age-adjusted suicide rate in the U.S. increased 24%, with the rate of increase greatest in girls aged 10-14 and men aged 45-64; the rate of male suicide is 3 times that for females.[12] One percent of U.S. adults suffers from schizophrenia.[13] It is estimated that about 47% of the U.S. adult population suffers from signs of an addictive disorder.[14]

Although about 90% of U.S. individuals get married before the age of 50, about 40% to 50% of married couples in the U.S. divorce.[15] In 2012, an estimated 686,000 U.S. children were victims of abuse: 78% neglected, 18% physically abused, 9% sexually abused, and 11% subjected to other types of abuse.[16]

More than one-third of U.S. adults is obese.[17] It is projected that by 2030, half of all adults (115 million adults) will be obese in the U.S..[18] Seventeen percent of U.S. children and adolescents are obese.[19] Between the 1970s and 2008, the prevalence of obesity in the U.S. doubled for children aged 2-5 years, quadrupled for children aged 6-11 years, tripled for children aged 12-19 years, and doubled for adults.[20]

U.S. children spend more than seven and a half hours daily in front of a TV, video-game, or computer screen, and only one in three children engages in physical activity every day.[21] More than 80% of adolescents do not meet guidelines for aerobic activity for youth, and more than 80% of adults do not do recommended amounts of aerobic and strength training.[22]

Humans have driven many lands to desertification by stripping lands of trees and vegetation, intensive farming, and overgrazing animals. World-wide, about 52% of agricultural land is moderately to severely degraded, affecting 1.5 billion people.[23] Every year, 12 million hectares of cropland – which could produce 20 million tons of grain – is lost to drought and desertification.[24] Land degradation directly affects 74% of the world's impoverished people.[25] Modern intensive mono-crop agriculture has rapidly degraded topsoil, and if current rates of soil loss continue, all of the world's top soil could be gone by 2076.[26]

Since 1900, the U.S.A. has depleted about 1,000 cubic kilometers (264 trillion gallons) of water from underground aquifers.[27] Agricultural fertilizer run-off has created dead zones devoid of animal life in many areas of the U.S. – especially along the East Coast, in the Great Lakes, and the Gulf of Mexico which has the second largest dead zone in the world.[28]

Globalization is introducing invasive plant, animal, and pathogen species into Africa and Asia, and these threaten biodiversity and the economies, livelihoods and health of people across the world, especially those in the poorest nations which have the least capacity to deal with them.[29] International "free trade" has introduced very destructive invasive species into U.S. forests[30] and these have "significantly impacted United States ecosystems and cost millions of dollars to prevent, detect and control."[31]

Two centuries of free trade has also introduced at least 25 invasive fish species and 7 invasive plant species into the Great Lakes, damaging the economy and health of people who rely on those lake for food and water.[32] More than 30 foreign invasive insects – including the Africanized Honeybee, Asian Tiger Mosquito, Mediterranean Fruit Fly, and the Fire Ant – and 4 invasive vertebrates are harming U.S. ecosystems, agriculture and people.[33] Invasive species are also having a destructive effect on European ecosystems.[34]

The social and religious traditions that inspired people for millennia have lost their influence on humanity. In modernized nations, family, community and national traditions have come under attack and are on the verge of extinction.

These are just some of the more prominent signs that our modern way of life is way off balance. We are witnessing the physical, mental, and moral degeneration of humanity and the destruction of the natural resources on which we depend for our lives. It is clear that we do not understand the Order of the Universe.

Who can save us? Many people hope that "experts" will take care of the problems, but we must realize that these problems are results of our own daily thoughts, words and deeds. In THE GREAT LEARNING,[35] Confucius wrote:

> "The ancients who wished to illustrate illustrious virtue throughout the kingdom, first ordered well their own states. Wishing to order well their states, they first regulated their families. Wishing to regulate their families, they first cultivated their persons. Wishing to cultivate their persons, they first rectified their hearts. Wishing to rectify their hearts, they first sought to be sincere in their thoughts. Wishing to be sincere in their thoughts, they first extended to the

utmost their knowledge. Such extension of knowledge lay in the investigation of things.

"Things being investigated, knowledge became complete. Their knowledge being complete, their thoughts were sincere. Their thoughts being sincere, their hearts were then rectified. Their hearts being rectified, their persons were cultivated. Their persons being cultivated, their families were regulated. Their families being regulated, their states were rightly governed. Their states being rightly governed, the whole kingdom was made tranquil and happy.

"From the Son of Heaven down to the mass of the people, all must consider the cultivation of the person the root of everything besides."

You are at the root of everything. Every day the average person consumes 3-5 pounds of food. Your diet determines your own physical and mental health more than any other single factor in your control, and it also primarily determines your impact on natural resources.

Through your thoughts, words and deeds, including especially your food choices, you control your mind and body and your impact on your family, community, nation, and Nature. By changing your daily thoughts, words, deeds, and diet, you will improve yourself and develop to your full potential, and also create a more harmonious relationship with Nature.

Starting with regeneration of your blood and the cells of your body and brain, then proceeding to develop your full physical, mental, and moral potential, you will inspire changes in your family and community. By being "The One" you are waiting for, you can do everything in your power to reverse the degeneration of humanity and Nature.

You can create a healthier world by becoming a healthier human.

NOTES

[1] CDC, NCHHSTP Newsroom, "2015 STD Surveillance Report Press Release."
<https://www.cdc.gov/nchhstp/newsroom/2016/std-surveillance-report-2015-press-release.html>

[2] Mermin J, "Have STDs Reach Crisis Level? The Status Quo Is No Longer Enough," Huffington Post 2016 Oct 20.
<http://www.huffingtonpost.com/dr-jonathan-mermin/have-stds-reached-crisis_b_12577246.html>

[3] CDC, "Birth Defects: Data & Statistics."
<http://www.cdc.gov/ncbddd/birthdefects/data.html>

[4] NIH, Nation Institute of Dental and Craniofacial Research, "Find Data by Topic." <http://www.nidcr.nih.gov/DataStatistics/FindDataByTopic/>

[5] NIH, National Institute of Diabetes and Digestive and Kidney Diseases, "Digestive Diseases Statistics for the United States."
<https://www.niddk.nih.gov/health-information/health-statistics/Pages/digestive-diseases-statistics-for-the-united-states.aspx>

[6] CDC, "Diabetes Home: 2014 National Diabetes Statistics Report."
<http://www.cdc.gov/diabetes/data/statistics/2014statisticsreport.html>

[7] American Heart Association, "New statistics show one of every three U.S. deaths caused by cardiovascular disease."
<http://newsroom.heart.org/news/new-statistics-show-one-of-every-three-u-s-deaths-caused-by-cardiovascular-disease>

[8] American Cancer Society, Cancer Statistics Center. <https://cancerstatisticscenter.cancer.org/?_ga=1.232068575.1792849541.1478892116#/>

[9] Dooley MA, Hogan SL, "Environmental Epidemiology and Risk Factors for Autoimmune Disease," Current Opinion in Rheumatology 2003;15(2). <http://www.medscape.com/viewarticle/449854>

[10] Barrocas, Andrea L. et al. "Rates of Nonsuicidal Self-Injury in Youth: Age, Sex, and Behavioral Methods in a Community Sample." *Pediatrics* 130.1 (2012): 39–45. *PMC*. Web. 11 Nov. 2016.

[11] NIH, National Institute of Mental Health, "Major Depression Among Adults." <https://www.nimh.nih.gov/health/statistics/prevalence/major-depression-among-adults.shtml>

[12] CDC National Center for Health Statistics, "Increase in Suicide in the United States, 1999-2014." <http://www.cdc.gov/nchs/products/databriefs/db241.htm>

[13] NIH, National Institute of Mental Health, ""Schizophrenia." <https://www.nimh.nih.gov/health/statistics/prevalence/schizophrenia.shtml>

[14] Sussman, Steve, Nadra Lisha, and Mark Griffiths. "Prevalence of the Addictions: A Problem of the Majority or the Minority?" *Evaluation & the health professions* 34.1 (2011): 3–56. *PMC*. Web. 12 Nov. 2016. <https://www.ncbi.nlm.nih.gov/pmc/articles/PMC3134413/>

[15] American Psychological Association, "Marriag & Divorce." <http://www.apa.org/topics/divorce/>

[16] CDC, "Child Maltreatment: Facts at a Glance, 2014." <http://www.cdc.gov/violenceprevention/pdf/childmaltreatment-facts-at-a-glance.pdf>

[17] CDC, "Overweight & Obesity." <https://www.cdc.gov/obesity/data/adult.html>

[18] President's Council on Fitness, Sports & Nutrition, "Facts & Statistics." <http://www.fitness.gov/resource-center/facts-and-statistics/>

[19] Ibid.

[20] Ibid.

[21] Ibid.

[22] Ibid.

[23] UN, "Desertification." <http://www.un.org/en/events/desertificationday/background.shtml>

[24] Ibid.

[25] Ibid.

[26] Arsenault C, "Only 60 Years of Farming Left If Soil Degradation Continues," Scientific American 2016. <https://www.scientificamerican.com/article/only-60-years-of-farming-left-if-soil-degradation-continues/>

[27] Konkow LF, "Groundwater Depletion in the United States," USGS Scientific Investigations Report 2013-5079, 63p., <http://pubs.usgs.gov/sir/2013/5079> (Available only online.)

[28] National Ocean Service, "What is a dead zone?" <http://oceanservice.noaa.gov/facts/deadzone.html>

[29] Early, Regan et al. "Global Threats from Invasive Alien Species in the Twenty-First Century and National Response Capacities." *Nature Communications* 7 (2016): 12485. *PMC*. Web. 12 Nov. 2016. <https://www.ncbi.nlm.nih.gov/pmc/articles/PMC4996970/>

[30] USDA, Forest Service, "Identifying & Preventing Invasive Species Threats." <http://www.fs.fed.us/research/invasive-species/prevention/>

[31] USDA Forest Service, "Invasive Species." <http://www.fs.fed.us/research/invasive-species/>

[32] EPA, "Invasive Species in the Great Lakes."
<https://www.epa.gov/greatlakes/invasive-species-great-lakes>

[33] USDA National Invasive Species Information Center > Animals.
<https://www.invasivespeciesinfo.gov/animals/main.shtml>

[34] USDA National Invasive Species Information Center > International > Europe.
<https://www.invasivespeciesinfo.gov/international/europe.shtml>

[35] Confucius. The Great Learning.
<http://classics.mit.edu/Confucius/learning.html>

1: MACROBIOTIC MINDSET

The word "macrobiotic" was coined by the eminent German physician Christoph Wilhelm Hufeland (1762-1836) to refer to the art and science of promoting health and prolonging life.[1] It comes from the Greek *makrobiotikos*, meaning "long-lived," or "great life." The word "diet" is derived from the Greek *diaita* which means "way of life." The phrase "macrobiotic diet" literally means "long-life way" and "great life way."

These days, many people think that proper nutrition and physical fitness are the essential keys to health and longevity. In contrast, Hufeland found that while these may be sufficient for health of animals, human health depends also on adherence to high moral standards. In his words:

> "I have found more than once, in the course of my labor, that the physical man cannot be separated from his higher moral object: and I may, perhaps, reckon it a small merit in the present performance, that it will not only establish the truth and heighten the value of the moral laws, in the eyes of many, by showing that they are indispensably necessary for the physical support and prolongation of life but that it demonstrates, that the physical nature of man has been suited to his higher moral destination; that this makes an essential difference between the nature of man and the nature of animals; that without moral cultivation man is in continual contradiction with his own nature; and that, by culture alone, he becomes even physically perfect. May I be so fortunate, by these means, as to accomplish two objects: not only to render the life of man more healthful and longer; but

also, by exciting his exertions for that purpose, to make him better and more virtuous! I can at any rate assert, that man will in vain seek for the one without the other, and that physical and moral health are as nearly related as the body and the soul. They flow from the same sources ; become blended together ; and when united, the result is, HUMAN NATURE ENNOBLED AND RAISED TO PERFECTION." [2]

These words of Hufeland resonate with those of many physicians, philosophers and sages who have since ancient times taught that humans have a divine destiny that every individual can realize through complete self-cultivation. For ages the sages have identified five main aims for seekers of a great life:

- Material prosperity acquired through expressing one's unique talents and gifts in noble occupations.
- Enjoyment of natural pleasures such as family, play, sports, art, music, sex, and nature's beauty and grandeur.
- Virtue and honor acquired by integrity and alignment of thought, word, and deed with Natural Moral Law.
- Self-mastery and realization of one's full physical, mental, and moral potential.
- Liberation from ignorance and bondage.

In my view, this is macrobiotics: the art of creating a noble, great life through self-realization of your physical, mental, moral, and spiritual potential.

You are to realize this potential in this very life, and through self-cultivation you will influence the destiny of your family, community and nation. A great soul leaves a legacy that inspires others to greatness. You can achieve immortality through the legacy of your words and deeds. This is about being an inspiration, not necessarily about being famous.

> Cattle die, kinsmen die, and so must one die oneself.
> But one thing I know which never dies –
> the fame of a dead man's deeds.
>
> THE HÁVAMÁL
> Verse 76
>
> To die, but not be forgotten, is to be immortal.
>
> TAO TE CHING
> Chapter 33

After the body dies, one lives on in the memory of others. You will likely be forgotten unless you live a great life consisting of actions and contributions that people want to remember because it gives them joy to do so.

You only have limited time. Use it to make your life great.

SELF RESPONSIBILITY

Epictetus was born a slave in the Roman Empire about 55 A.D.. He was crippled, but he discovered a passion for philosophy in youth, and he got permission from his owner Epaphroditos to study Stoic philosophy under the master Gaius Musonius Rufus. Rufus advocated a simple vegetarian diet and a minimalist lifestyle as part of the philosopher's essential quest to develop of good character, a sound mind, and a tough, healthy body. Epictetus obtained his liberation from slavery after the cruel, tyrannical Roman emperor Nero died in 63 A.D.

Some time after this, Epictetus began to teach philosophy. In 93 A.D. the emperor Domitian banned philosophers from Rome, so Epictetus moved to Greece where he established a school of Stoic philosophy. One of his students was Marcus Aurelius, who went on to become the emperor of Rome. Though born a "slave" he made himself into a great man, remembered and revered to this day, by taking control of himself, accepting and yet rising above his accidental circumstances.

Epictetus taught that if you are unhappy, it is your own fault. Though born a "slave" he made himself into a great man, remembered and revered to this day, by taking control of himself and rising above his accidental circumstances.

Epictetus taught that slavery consists of trying to control things outside of oneself – possessions, status, power – but failing to control things that are in one's power: one's thoughts, opinions, impulses, desires, aversions, words and deeds.

In THE GREAT LEARNING, Confucius taught that a man who wants to change the world starts by rectifying himself. The man who makes himself strong and healthy will make his family strong and healthy; when the family is strong and healthy the community will become strong and healthy; and when the community becomes strong and healthy, the nation becomes strong and healthy. Self-cultivation is the root of a healthy world.

This world is full of beauty and opportunity. If you are not happy, if you have not attained your potential, take responsibility. Blaming others makes you a slave to things beyond your control.

You are the one you have been waiting for.

> To accuse others for one's own misfortunes is a sign of want of education. To accuse oneself shows that one's education has begun. To accuse neither oneself nor others shows that one's education is complete.
>
> Epictetus

SELF-RELIANCE

Find the resources you need within yourself instead of seeking to take them from others. Also, when you give help to others, do your best to help them become self-reliant rather than dependent on your help. Cultivate independence in yourself and in others.

SELF-DISCIPLINE

Weak, unhappy and unhealthy people want to control things that are beyond them. They want others to change. They want the world to change. They want the weather to change.

If you want to be strong, happy and healthy, focus on developing control over what you can control: your own thoughts, words, and deeds. Forget about trying to control other people, the world, or the weather.

True strength comes from conquering one's own weaknesses and vices. Stop examining others and start examining your own life. Pay attention to your thoughts, words, and deeds. Find your own faults, vices and weakness and route them out.

> For a person who is not aware that he is doing anything wrong has no desire to be put right. You have to catch yourself doing it before you can reform. Some people boast about their failings; can you imagine someone who counts his faults as merits ever giving thought to their cure? So— to the best of your ability—demonstrate your own guilt, conduct inquiries of your own into all the evidence against yourself. Play the first part of prosecutor, then of judge and finally of pleader in mitigation. Be harsh with yourself at times.
>
> Seneca
> LETTERS FROM A STOIC

HONESTY

Dishonest people live in conflict with Reality, which makes them sick, weak, vulnerable and untrustworthy. When you align your thoughts, words, and deeds with Reality, you will have Reality supporting rather than opposing you. *You can't be healthy if you are habitually dishonest.*

To enjoy surfing, surfers align themselves with the tide of the ocean so that it can propel them more powerfully than they can achieve on their own. Similarly, to create a great life, you must align your thoughts, words and deeds with Nature and Life, so that it can propel you farther than you could manage on your own.

The positive practice of honesty includes not telling lies, associating with and praising honest people, teaching children to be honest, keeping promises and appointments, actively revealing truth (that which can't be denied), dispelling superstitions, and distinguishing hypotheses from truth. The honest person also disapproves of, dislikes, despises and avoids association with dishonest people, does not like stories of cheating, and denounces those who lie and cheat. An honest person tells the truth because it is the right thing to do, and avoids doing dishonest things just because they are dishonest.

AUSTERITY

Austerity is the ability to bear hardship for a noble purpose. Any honorable path will present difficulties. Without austerity, one will give up the moment any hardships arise.

Moreover, one should seek and embrace hardship because it activates latent potentials. A very comfortable life leads to weakness and unhappiness of body and mind. As the Roman poet Horace wrote, "Adversity elicits talents which in easy circumstances would have lain dormant."

> Suffering! We owe to it all that is good in us, all that gives value to life; we owe to it pity, we owe to it courage, we owe to it all the virtues.
>
> Anatole France

Do not complain about adversaries, but recognize them as valuable friends. George Ohsawa wrote "A strong cruel enemy is particularly valuable; without him, one becomes idle, weak, and stupid." As Nietzsche famously wrote, "That which does not kill me makes me stronger." This expresses the spirit of a person who accepts adversity as necessary and beneficial to development of personal power.

MINDFULNESS OF MORTALITY

Realize that your time is limited. You have no idea how long you have to live. Will you spend your time wisely, or will you die with regrets? What will be the legacy of your life? Make it great.

> Not to live as if you had endless years ahead of you. Death overshadows you. While you're alive and able – be good.
>
> Marcus Aurelius
> MEDITATIONS

APPRECIATION

A healthy person has deep appreciation for the gift of life and the wonders of nature.

> Your appearance, voice, behavior, and even your criticism should distribute deep gratitude to all in your presence. All your words should be expressive of a deep gratitude, like the singing of birds and insects or the poems of Tagore. The stars, the sun, the mountains, rivers, and seas are all ours. How can we exist without being happy? We should be full of delight like a boy who has just received a magnificent present. If we are not, we lack good health and good humor.
>
> George Ohsawa

Focus your attention on what you have, not on what you don't have. When you focus on what you don't have, you drag yourself into poverty. When you focus on what you do have, you make yourself wealthy.

PURPOSEFULNESS

You need a deep sense of purpose. You need to know why you exist and what you want to accomplish. You need to know what you stand for, and what you will stand against.

You can live a small life, devoted to your own comfort, or you can live a great life devoted to realization of your full physical, mental, and moral potential while helping and inspire others.

What is your noble purpose? *Its time for you find it.* Here are some ideas to get you thinking:

- Dispelling myths and spreading truth.
- Raising healthy and strong children.
- Providing healthy foods for other people (e.g. farming).
- Helping others develop independence in food, shelter, etc..
- Helping others achieve physical fitness.
- Protecting people from crime.
- Teaching others how to defend themselves.
- Protecting natural resources for future generations.
- Building healthy, non-toxic homes.
- Crafting natural homes and furnishings
- Crafting natural fiber clothing
- Creating techniques for capturing or generating non-polluting energy.
- Providing natural health care.

- Providing education aimed at preserving and expanding accumulated traditional knowledge, promoting healthy, righteous lifestyles, and improving people's judgement.

To maintain your purpose-oriented mindset, you can use a daily statement of purpose. If you don't have a purpose statement already, create one now. Write down what you want to do, why it is important to you to do it, and how you will help others by fulfilling your purpose.

GENEROSITY

The Universe has given you your unique life, body, mind and the whole world to enjoy. The Universe produces and offers to you everything you need: water, food, air, plants, animals, minerals. Your parents gave you life and fed you. You have eaten many plants and animals to keep yourself alive.

How can you repay this gift? Return the favor. You have been given physical and mental gifts and talents. It is your responsibility to develop these talents and gifts and use them to help others become healthy, strong, and wise.

COURAGE

Courage comes from the Latin word for "heart." To manifest courage means to *care enough to speak or act* in alignment with Truth and Virtue, even if it entails some danger to yourself. For example, speak or stand up for what you know is right, or against what is wrong, even if you would be more comfortable not doing so, and in spite of any fear you may feel. Note that bravery does not require stupidity. For example, if you see someone in danger but know that you don't have the ability to help them without getting hurt yourself – e.g. someone is drowning but you don't know how to swim – you use courage to get help. Simply, *courage means converting care into righteous action.*

HOSPITALITY

Hospitality means being friendly, welcoming and generous to kindred, friends, and cordial travelers. There is no virtue in extending hospitality to hostile people who want only to harm or take things from you. It is necessary to temper hospitality with good judgement.

DILIGENCE

Anyone who wishes to prosper must be diligent in both work and play. Whenever you work, do your best, and always aim to get the most results possible from the time and effort you invest. Use your time and energy wisely and productively. Do work that produces useful goods and services, train yourself to produce physical fitness, and learn things to upgrade your knowledge and skill. Also, when you play, immerse yourself fully into the game or pastime to get as much fun and joy as can be gotten from it.

PERSEVERANCE

A Japanese proverb states: "Fall down nine times, get up ten." The I CHING (BOOK OF CHANGES) frequently advises "Perseverance furthers." Simply, if your work is righteous, despite all obstacles, do not give up! You can't live on this plane without encountering obstacles in your path. If you want a great life, you must persevere in spite of obstacles.

LOVE OF NATURE

The Universe is the Creator of all things. Through division, separation, individuation, development and evolution It strives to self-realize all of Its infinite potential. Every one of Nature's forces, laws, elements and creatures is an expression of the divine and sacred Universe.

You yourself are an offspring of Nature. The Creator lives in, through, and as you. You are composed of Nature's elements and sustained by air, water, soil, sun, moon, plants and animals. To be healthy and strong, love Nature as you would love a parent who has nurtured and protected you. The way to love Nature is to enjoy her gifts and obey her Laws of Life.

> Life in all its fullness is Mother Nature obeyed.
>
> Weston Price
> NUTRITION AND PHYSICAL DEGENERATION

NON-CREDO

Liberate yourself from commercial media programs (e.g. radio, television, newspapers, magazines, etc.) which are designed to program you to think and act in ways that serve the owners of those outlets.

The pursuit of truth and process of self-realization is largely a process of discarding false ideas and beliefs about oneself and Reality that we received from ignorant, misinformed, or power- or profit-seeking people (public schools, media, politicians, corporations, etc.) who benefit from the ignorance and enslavement of others.

> In the pursuit of learning, every day something is acquired.
> In the pursuit of TAO, every day something is dropped.
>
> TAO TE CHING
> Chapter 48

Do not blindly believe what others have told you, but discover truth for yourself. Use your free time to learn by reading books and other educational materials, or study yourself, nature and the world around you through direct experience.

Do not send your children to public schools. The powers that be use public schools to program children to become drones (slaves) for their purposes. Choose home schooling or alternative schools. Generally home schooling is best as it strengthens the bond between parents and children.

SURRENDER

Nature and human events have their own cycles and rhythms which are beyond anyone's control. Learn to trust and ride these waves.

By trusting Tao, the Infinite Universe, you can release yourself from worry, doubt, and fear and realize peace of mind. When you trust Tao, Tao will trust you.

> Forget about controlling what happens; learn to wish that everything that happens happens just as it happens. Then…all will go exactly as planned.
>
> Epictetus
> HANDBOOK, 8

NON-AGGRESSION

Do not *initiate* violence against other people. Follow the Golden Rule: *Do not do to others what one does not want done to oneself.* This Rule is called Golden because adherence to it brings every One all Good – health, happiness, liberty, and prosperity. Violation of this Rule – simply, taking Life, Liberty, or Property from innocents – in a word, theft – produces illness, unhappiness, disorder, slavery, and poverty.

However, it is very important to note that the non-aggression principle does not proscribe self-defense. The Golden Rule does not prescribe "turning the other cheek" or "loving" people who spitefully use, persecute and injure you or others. Confucius advocated living by the Golden Rule, but he also said:

> If one repays evil with good, what then will you return for good? Return good for good, and repay evil with justice.
>
> Confucius

To manifest a high level of judgement one must take a big view of things. Criminals declare by their actions that they are a threat to the well-being of one's family, tribe and nation and do not deserve kindness or consideration. Protecting criminals puts innocent members of your family, tribe, and nation at risk of injury. Letting a criminal loose means doing harm to many other people. Often it is necessary to injure and disable a criminal or predator in order to do for others what you would want them to do for you.

If you are sentimentally "kind" people you influence will just become weak and vulnerable. If you want to make people strong and confident, one must sometimes be tough, harsh and demanding. However, you may not demand of others what you do not demand of yourself.

GOOD JUDGEMENT

To become healthy and strong and realize your full potential you need the ability to distinguish between natural and artificial, true and false, right and wrong, real and unreal. We call this ability *judgement*.

Whereas materialistic medicine considers skin barriers and white blood cells to be the front line of the immune system, macrobiotic philosophy identifies judgement as the first responder. White blood cells can respond to a pathogenic influence only after it enters the body. Through judgement one decides what and who one will allow into one's inner sanctum through food, vision, hearing, odors, conversation, information, and sexual contact.

Poor judgement leads to unhealthy choices, allowing harmful influences into the Temple of One Self, producing misery and disorders of body and mind. Good judgement makes healthy choices, rejecting poison and only allowing beneficial influences to enter the Temple of One Self, producing health and happiness.

Your success depends on your level of judgement. It is your responsibility to improve your judgement. No one can do it for you. George Ohsawa identified seven levels of judgement, as follows[3]:

1. *Mechanical*: Your actions are mindless, random and automatic reactions to internal and external events.
2. *Sensory*: You pursue momentary pleasure and avoids momentary pain.
3. *Sentimental*: You make choices based on emotions, social acceptance, aesthetics and nostalgia.
4. *Intellectual*: You use only reason, logic, and current scientific concepts and theories to make choices.
5. *Moral*: You know the objective difference between right and wrong and use moral principles to make choices.
6. *Metaphysical*: You seek to distinguish between temporary and eternal truths.
7. *Universal*: Your thoughts, words and deeds are aligned with Reality and Natural Law. You enact excellence and magnificence without even trying or noticing.

To raise your level of judgement, you have to learn from others and from experience. You have to welcome difficulties and challenges and work your way through them. You have to learn from people who have developed a high level of judgement. It helps to study philosophy, metaphysics, and ethics. Most of all, you must have a goal to gain wisdom.

> Cultivate Virtue in your self,
> And Virtue will be real.
> Cultivate it in the family,
> And Virtue will abound.
> Cultivate it in the village,
> And Virtue will grow.
> Cultivate it in the nation,
> And Virtue will be abundant.
> Cultivate it in the Universe,
> And Virtue will be everywhere.
>
> TAO TE CHING
> Chapter 54

NOTES

[1] Hufeland CW. *Art of Prolonging Life*, ed. by Erasmus Wilson, F.R.S. (Boston: Ticknor, Reed, and Fields, 1854).

[2] Hufeland CW. *Art of Prolonging Life*, ed. by Erasmus Wilson, F.R.S. (Boston: Ticknor, Reed, and Fields, 1854). <https://archive.org/stream/hufelandsartofpr00huferich/hufelandsartofpr00huferich_djvu.txt>

[3] My presentation of levels 1-5 and 7 follows George Ohsawa, but we differ on level 6, which he called "Ideological" referring to religious ideologies. Conventional religious doctrines generally mix a mistaken belief in "authority (over others)" with judgement levels 1-6. Pure level 6 is generally only reached by philosophers. One at level 7 is a sage.

2: NATURAL LAW

> Look, it cannot be seen - it is beyond form.
> Listen, it cannot be heard - it is beyond sound.
> Grasp, it cannot be held - it is intangible.
> These three are indefinable;
> Therefore they are joined in one.
> From above it is not bright;
> From below it is not dark:
> An unbroken thread beyond description.
> It returns to nothingness.
> The form of the formless,
> The image of the imageless,
> It is called indefinable and beyond imagination.
> Stand before it and there is no beginning.
> Follow it and there is no end.
> Stay with the ancient Tao,
> Move with the present.
> Knowing the ancient beginning is the essence of Tao.
>
> TAO TE CHING
> Chapter 14

THE UNIVERSE

Nothing exists outside of Reality. All things are temporary manifestations of one Reality, which we call the Universe.

The Universe is perpetually changing in an orderly procession according to Natural Laws. Those who understand and align their thoughts, words, and deeds with Natural Laws survive and prosper. They are like surfers who align themselves with the tide of the ocean so that it can propel them more powerfully than they can achieve on their own.

Those who do not understand or rebel against Natural Laws are destroyed. They are like surfers who try to go opposite to the tides. Reality will crush them. Physical, mental, and social disorder, disease, disintegration, dissolution all result from thought, words and deeds that do not align with Natural Law, the Order of the Universe.

> Heaven and Earth are impartial;
> They see the ten thousand things as straw dogs.
> The wise are impartial;
> They see the people as straw dogs.
>
> TAO TE CHING
> Chapter Five

Individuals, families, clans, tribes, and nations that align their thoughts, words, and deeds with Natural Law prosper in the short and long term. Those that do not, may prosper in the short term, but in the long term they will disappear.

People tend to ignore Natural Law, or make futile attempts to circumvent it. We have a tendency to perceive hardships, sickness, accidents, and other unpleasant experiences as unfair and unjust. This is due to our limited perspectives. In Reality, nothing is unfair or unjust.

Since all events occur according to Natural Laws of cause and effect, action and consequences, we can not create any lasting good unless we understand and harmonize our actions with Human Nature and Natural Law.

Four Principles of Natural Law

1. All things are unique temporary expressions of the Infinite Universe; no two things are identical.
2. Every thing changes; no thing is permanent.
3. All things have both a front and a back, proportional to one another.
4. Opposites are complementary.

Yin and Yang

Since all beings are expressions of One Ultimate Reality, all opposites are complementary aspects of One. The One can never be divided against Itself; Reality never contradicts Itself.

Whenever you evenly divide any One into two, the result will always be two complementary halves which mirror one another. It is impossible to divide One into two with any other result. Since each half of The One lacks what occurs in the other half, each is incomplete without the other. Chinese scientists illustrated this fact with the classic yin-yang symbol (which is a representation of the graph obtained by plotting on a compass the lengths and positions of the shadows cast at noon, day after day for an entire year, by a pole posted at right angles to ground).[1]

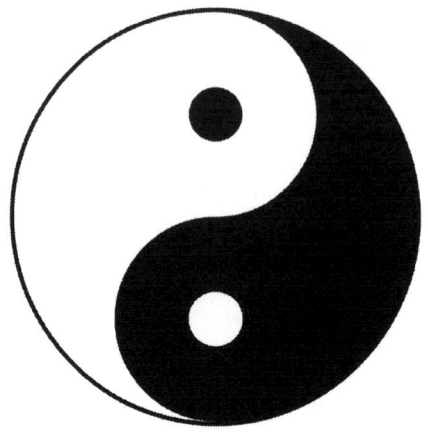

The circle represents The One, which in Chinese science is called TAO. The two halves represent what happens when The One appears as if two: Each side is a mirror image of and dependent upon the other for expression of its own nature. For example, male and female are complementary opposites, each of which depends on the other for its identity and expression. Just as a mountain can't exist without a valley, male can't exist without female, nor female without male. The two are mutually interdependent, co-created, and co-creative. The same applies to Seer/seen, inside/outside, male/female, hot/cold, old/young, wet/dry, self/other, electron/proton, high/low, strong/weak, parents/children.

In ignorance of the Unity in duality, many people have valued one of expression of Reality over the other. For example, some people think that the masculine expression of Reality (TAO) is bad and should be eliminated, in favor of the feminine expression (or vice versa). But if you eliminate the masculine, you will simultaneously eliminate the feminine (and vice versa).

The following table displays the sensible characteristics of each pole of expression.

Characteristic	Yang	Yin
Emblem	Fire	Water
Entity	Energy / Pattern	Matter
Colors	Bright Red, yellow, orange, white, brown	Dark Green, blue, black, purple
Sound	Loud	Quiet
Odor	Strong, pungent	Faint, floral
Taste	Salty, bland, pungent	Sweet, sour, bitter
Texture	Hard, rough, dry	Soft, smooth, moist
Dimension	Time	Space
Form	Contracted, compact, hard	Expanded, loose, fragile
Function	Fusion Assimilation Gathering Organization	Diffusion Dispersion Separation Decomposition
Movement	More active, faster	Less active, slower
Vibration	Long wave, low frequency	Short wave, high frequency
Direction	Downward Centripetal	Upward Centrifugal
Position	Inside, central	Outside, peripheral

Characteristic	Yang	Yin
Density	High	Low
Temperature	Higher	Lower
Climate	Hot, dry	Cold, humid
Biology	Animal	Vegetable
Sex	Male	Female
Attitude	Positive	Negative
Work	Physical or social	Mental, private

Nine Natural Laws of Change

Yin and yang phenomena interact in an orderly fashion, according to the following laws of change:

1. THE ONE expresses Itself in a continuous evolutionary motion of two complementary polarities: yin and yang.
2. Yin moves centrifugally, yang moves centripetally, together creating energy and all phenomena.
3. Opposites attract one another and likes repel one another.
4. The strength of attraction or repulsion always represents the degree of difference or similarity between them.
5. Yin and yang combine in an infinite variety of proportions, creating an infinite variety of unique phenomena.
6. Nothing is absolutely yin or yang. Everything arises from and includes interaction of both forces.
7. No thing is neutral; always either yin or yang characteristics dominate.

8. Great yin attracts small yin. Great yang attracts small yang.
9. At the extreme point, yin reverts to yang, or vice versa.

ULTIMATE REALITY: AWARENESS

If one fails to distinguish between *Presence* and *existence*, one can get very confused about the ultimate nature of Reality, particularly if one has received a high degree of indoctrination in "scientific" materialism.

It is possible to imagine the absence of any particular thing, as well as the sum total of things – the world, all phenomena. Indeed, the perennial human quest to understand the origin of things, and the world, arises directly from our ability to imagine the absence of things. Our ability to imagine the absence of all *things* gives rise to our questions "Where did this world come from?" and "Why is there something, rather than nothing?"

Since we can imagine the absence of any particular *thing* as well as the absence of the world (all things), it follows that we directly perceive that no *thing* or *collection of things* is ultimately Real. Things are only phenomena, temporary "reality."

Individuals with different sensory and cognitive equipment live in one Reality but different worlds. Dogs, cats, bumble bees, and humans all exist in one Reality, but due to differences in sensory and cognitive equipment, each species experiences a somewhat different world than the others. For example, most humans live in a very colorful world, but dogs and cats do not perceive colors seen by humans. On the other hand, dogs and cats hear and smell many things humans do not hear and smell.

What any individual human sees, hears, tastes, smells, or hears depends on the condition of his sense organs, his perspective, and, to some extent, his conceptual framework (beliefs). For example, color-blind people do not see exactly the same world as those who are not color blind. Women see things somewhat differently from men; people from different cultures have different perceptions and experience different phenomena. Hence, one's world is an appearance, a temporary reality, not *ultimate* Reality.

Since beliefs can condition our perceptions, one must suspend commitment to one's beliefs in order to view Reality. This means shifting from thinking and imagination to paying attention to your direct experience, which is known as phenomenology and empiricism.

Ultimate Reality is That, the Presence of which no one can deny. Is there any Presence that in direct experience no one can doubt or deny? Indeed, there is.

No one can deny the Presence of Awareness because It must be Present before any denial can be made or detected. If anyone were to make the statement "Awareness is not present" or the equivalent "I am not present" he would be involved in a phenomenological Self-contradiction because only one who is aware can make such a statement.

Further, it is impossible to imagine the absence of Awareness, because Awareness is required to exercise imagination. Any effort to imagine the absence of Awareness only confirms its Presence. Similarly, it is impossible to imagine the absence of imagination, or to think away thought. I invite you to try.

The word "exist" comes from the Latin *existere* which means "to step out, stand forth, emerge, appear; exist, be." Awareness, does not *ex-ist* because It does not "stand out" among other things in Reality. If one looks <u>out</u>ward, trying to find Awareness among things existing in Reality, one will never find or prove It, because It is the One looking!

Put pointedly, Awareness constitutes the One who looks outward, and is and must be Present ("pre-sent" means "before sense") before any *thing* can be known to exist. If you doubt, please try to produce an experience of any thing without Awareness being Present.

Now, try to describe Awareness. You will find that Awareness has no form, color, sound, texture, taste, or odor, although it is impossible to detect form, color, sound, texture, flavor, color or any other thing without Awareness.

Since Awareness has no form, it has no boundaries, i.e. It is Infinite and Eternal. Since It is not finite, it is not local; that is, it is ever Present, otherwise stated *omnipresent*.

Let me explain: One Awareness powers sentience in all sentient beings, in the same way that one ocean powers all waves, or one electrical force powers a myriad of different electrical phenomena and machines. Although a can opener and a computer may both be powered by electricity, each expresses the power of electricity in a different way due to specific construction. Between individual sentient beings, objects of Awareness differ, but the Seer of those objects is One. A chicken and a human differ in body constitution and location, so each experiences different things (sights, sounds, odors, flavors, textures), but that which powers their sentience is One. Thus, Awareness – also known as Spirit – is Universal.

It follows that One Awareness – that which we refer to when we say "I Am" – is the One Self of all sentient beings. Dear reader, It is your Nature, Origin, Source and Essence.

Thus, Awareness is that undeniable, formless Presence by which one knows oneself directly, and without which no experience or experiment can occur. Awareness empowers sentience, and detects, affirms and proves the existence of things. If you doubt the latter, attempt to prove the existence of something without the Presence of Awareness. You will quickly find that no "proof" can occur without the Presence of Awareness.

> Knowing others constitutes wisdom;
> Knowing One Self constitutes enlightenment.
> Mastering others requires force;
> Mastering oneself needs strength.
> One who embraces contentment remains rich.
> Perseverance signifies willpower.
> One who remains present endures.
> In eternal Presence one dies but the One does not perish.
>
> TAO TE CHING
> Chapter 33

Since Ultimate Reality is that, the Presence of which can't be denied or contradicted by any thing or any One at any time or place, and no One can deny the Presence of Awareness at any time or place, it follows that Awareness – which I also call Spirit – is the Nature of Ultimate Reality, the Absolute, the Truth, the Eternal.

Put otherwise, since Reality is that which is ever Present, never absent, and Awareness is in our direct experience ever Present, never absent, it follows that the Ultimate Reality is Awareness.

Since Awareness is the Ultimate Reality, it follows that it is the back Ground and Source of all that is, i.e. the Universe. Indeed, Awareness *is* The One Turning Into The All (the literal meaning of "universe"). Put otherwise, the Knower is the Source of the Known. The material world unfolds from the immaterial Knower. Information precedes formation.

This is no "mystical" proposition. Throughout Nature, material forms unfold from seeds containing the information or knowledge-ability to generate the forms.

Thus, the Nature – the Source, Origin, and Essence – of Reality or the Universe is Awareness. The words Tao, Spirit, Awareness, The One, I Am, and most importantly, One Self, all refer to the One Abundant Infinite Eternal Presence that is the Nature, Source, Origin, and Essence of Reality.

To recap, Reality consists of Awareness which is:

- Undeniable.
- Ever Present, i.e. omnipresent and thus Eternal.
- The Source of all Powers, i.e. omnipotent.
- The Source of all Knowing, i.e. omniscient.
- The Origin of Intelligence and Intelligent Origin.
- The Source of Will, manifest in sentient beings.
- The Source of Life.
- Independent, Self-sufficient, Self-organizing.
- Absolutely free and sovereign.
- One unique Whole, i.e. an Individual.
- Complete and Perfect, not lacking anything.
- Abundant, plentiful, wealthy, inexhaustible, beauty-full.
- Generous and magnanimous, as it gives of Itself completely to generate and sustain all beings.

Body, Mind, Spirit

One Reality, our Universe, has three aspects:

- *Spirit*, which is pure Awareness, the Self-knowing Eternal and Infinite Presence. It is the Seer that can't be seen. It is the Causal Body, the Ultimate Creative Source of all powers and manifestations including Intelligence, Mind, Life, and Body. It manifests its boundlessness in Imagination which enables us to transcend temporary reality i.e. conditions.
- *Mind*, which is the power to receive and respond to ideas and impressions. Mind receives ideas from Spirit and through the Laws of Logic and Manifestation, Mind produces actions and conditions that manifest or realize the idea.
- *Body*, or Nature, which includes all material manifestations, and is the effect, result, or fruit of past thoughts, words, and deeds.

These three generate all things and experiences.

The Law of Return

In this Universe, every action has an equal and opposite reaction. Whatever you put out into the Universe, returns to you. Put otherwise, *as ye sow, so shall ye reap*.

Receipt of the natural consequences of one's actions is called *Natural Justice*. Natural Justice teaches us Natural Law.

Knowledge is Power

Human beings have a bipolar awareness or knowledge of external Reality and the internal Self.

Cultivating awareness of external Reality while engaging in trials and experiments leads to objective knowledge of Natural Laws of action and consequence (e.g. *As ye sow, so shall ye reap*), known as *science,* which enables us to reliably produce the goods we require (food, shelter, etc.).

Cultivation of Self-awareness leads to knowledge of the One Self and objective morality, known as *conscience.* Living in Self-awareness and alignment with Truth and Virtue is called Enlightenment.

Right and Wrong

Modern people are very confused about right and wrong. Thanks to indoctrination by "authorities" who profit from the people being ignorant of their own conscience and the objective difference between right and wrong, many people believe that right and wrong are "relative," a position known as moral relativism. In Reality, for humans, moral right and wrong are as objective as true and false in mathematics. It is no mistake that we use the word "right" as a synonym for both *true* and *moral*. The word is derived from the Latin *rectus* which means "straight, aligned, right." Most basically, it means *aligned with Reality.* Right action arises from *knowledge* of Reality, which is good or moral because it promotes life (survival, health, fitness, and reproduction).

The word "wrong" is derived from the Proto-Germanic *wrang* which means "crooked, wry, twisted." In other words, "wrong" means *not aligned with Reality.* That's why it is a synonym for *false* – "2 + 2 = 3" is wrong because it is false. Wrong action arises from ignorance of Reality, which is bad or immoral because it undermines life (survival, health, fitness, and reproduction). That is why the word *evil* – *live* spelled backwards – means harmful, bad, and immoral.

Table 2.1: Right vs. Wrong	
Right	**Wrong**
LATIN *rectus* "straight, aligned, right"	PROTO-GERMANIC *wrang* "crooked, wry, twisted"
ALIGNED WITH REALITY	*NOT* ALIGNED WITH REALITY
TRUE 2 + 2 = 4	FALSE 2 + 2 = 3
GOOD, MORAL	BAD, IMMORAL
PRO-LIFE	ANTI-LIFE

The Law of Property

Wrong action arises from ignorance of the Natural Law of Property or *ownership*. By Nature, right of command and use is determined by actual ownership. Ownership is defined as actual possession, command of, and authority for the property (body) in question. As a matter of fact one actually owns only that property which one can actually command and has obtained by one of the following three ways:

1. as a birth gift from Reality (i.e. one's mind and body, gifts and talent),
2. by labor transforming honestly acquired natural resources, or
3. by voluntary trade with another individual.

Wrong action occurs when someone uses force or fraud to take control of life, liberty, or property that by Natural Law belongs to another individual of your kind. Simply, it is aggression and theft. The principal forms of theft are:

- Taking life, known as murder.
- Taking bodily safety or integrity, known as assault.
- Taking liberty, known as threat, coercion or enslavement.
- Taking property, known as stealing or robbery.
- Taking truth or confidence, known as lying or fraud.
- Taking privacy, known as trespass, including sexual trespass, known as rape.
- Taking reputation, known as libel or defamation, often occurring during gossip.

Through self-reflection and conscience we all know these are wrong actions because we would not want them done to ourselves.

Those who practice aggression are called *unrighteous* because their actions are not-right-use of their property (body and mind). Aggression arises from faulty understanding, poor judgement and lack of alignment with Reality, which are faults and make one weak, so it is called *vice*. Wrong action produces personal and social disease, disorder, degeneration, corruption, bondage, slavery, and poverty.

Table 2.2: Right Action vs. Wrong Action	
RIGHT ACTION	**WRONG ACTION**
NON-AGGRESSION HARM-LESS TO OTHER'S PRIVATE PROPERTY	VIOLENCE, AGGRESSION HARM-FUL TO OTHER'S PRIVATE PROPERTY
RIGHT-USE RIGHTEOUS	NOT-RIGHT-USE UNRIGHTEOUS

Table 2.2: Right Action vs. Wrong Action	
RIGHT ACTION	**WRONG ACTION**
VIRTUE fr. LATIN virtus "strength, valor, courage"	VICE fr. LATIN vitium "fault, weakness, imperfection"
PERSONAL & SOCIAL FLOURISHING LIBERATION/LIBERTY HEALTH, FITNESS	PERSONAL & SOCIAL DEGENERATION BONDAGE/SLAVERY DISEASE, CORRUPTION

Right Action consists of right use of lawful property. Every one has the Natural Right to any action that does not infringe on any other individual's life, liberty, and honestly acquired property. Voluntary actions that generate goods and services that support and enhance life, liberty, health, happiness, and physical, mental, and spiritual prosperity for oneself, one's family, and one's community are right-use of one self. Those who enact Right Use are called *righteous*. Right Action brings strength, liberty, peace, and prosperity to a righteous individual or community. Hence it is called *virtue*.

FORCE, VIOLENCE, AND SELF-DEFENSE

Many people confuse force and violence, largely because people who profit from this confusion have deliberately created it by encouraging the use of the word "force" when the word "violence" should be used. Based on this confusion of the concepts of force and violence, many advocates of non-violence suggest that using force against aggressors is violence, as wrong as the aggression. I disagree.

The word "force" comes from the Latin *fortis* which means *strength*. All living beings must exert force in order to move, gather food, and sustain their lives and health. As I type this on my computer, I am exerting force against the keys on the keyboard, generating this document. If I talk or play any musical instrument, I must use force to generate the sounds. When I eat, I must exert force against the food in my mouth in order to chew it up, and my gastrointestinal tract will use force to propel the food through the system for digestion and assimilation. If I sit in meditation, I exert force to hold myself upright. People must properly use force to hug, shake hands, or engage in consensual loving sexual relations. If someone tries to harm me and I run away, I use force to do so. The appropriate use of force is required by and in alignment with Reality, therefore it is a right.

Table 2.3: Force vs. Violence	
Force	**Violence**
LATIN *fortis* "strength, power"	LATIN *violatio* "injury, irreverence, profanity"
To exert strength	To injure or damage someone
Support, enhance, or defend Life, Liberty, or Property	Initiated aggression and theft of Life, Liberty, or Property
Right	Wrong

The word "violence" comes from the Latin *violatio* which means *injury*. While it is true that one must use force in order to commit violence, an action is by Natural Law violent only if it injures someone through assault, robbery, libel, trespass, coercion, and other forms of theft listed above.

43

Nature gave all animals a natural impulse to use force in self-defense. By initiating an attempt to take life, liberty, or property that he does not rightly own, an aggressor violates the Order of the Universe, and is liable for damages he inflicts upon his target(s). A defendant has a Natural Right to protect his honestly acquired life, liberty and property, and thus is right ("has the right") to use as much force as necessary to stop the aggressor from doing injury or damage, up to and including deadly force, and this just use of force is *not* violence, it is *justice*.

To illustrate the last point: If Bob were to sneak upon and hit Joe and attempt to take his wallet, Bob would be committing an act of violence. If Joe strikes back at Bob, Joe is using defensive force and rendering justice, but he is not guilty of violence.

If two or more parties consent to an rule-bound temporary interaction that may result in bodily injury to some of the parties involved, none of the parties involved can be accused of violence unless rules are violated. For example, if Bob and Joe agreed to fight one another in a rule-bound boxing or mixed martial arts match, even though both parties will likely sustain injuries, the match is voluntary hence by Natural Law neither party is guilty of violence against the other, *unless* someone violates the rules agreed upon.

If you are unable to protect your self or a loved one from aggressors, someone's life or lineage may be cut short. Therefore, the study of martial arts – both unarmed and armed – is a part of practical macrobiotics, particularly for men.

NOTES

[1] Jaeger S. A Geomedical Approach to Chinese Medicine: The Origin of the Yin-Yang Symbol. In: Recent Advances in Theories and Practice of Chinese Medicine, ed. By Haixue Kuang. Intech, 2012

3: HEALTH & SICKNESS

> Health is a state of complete harmony of the body, mind and spirit. When one is free from physical disabilities and mental distractions, the gates of the soul open.
>
> B.K.S. Iyengar

HEALTH

The Oriental medicine concept of health markedly differs from the common idea of absence of immediately apparent disease or disorder. Health is not just the absence of overt disease; it is the full flowering of human potential in Body, Mind, and Spirit. Here are signs of health:

1. *Abundant energy.* A healthy person has abundant energy for accomplishment of his or her goals and dreams. In spite of whatever difficulties arise, a healthy person never complains of lacking energy to deal with them. A vital person never catches cold, no matter what the weather.

2. *Good appetite*: Good appetite includes a healthy appetite for simple natural foods, play, work, sex, and life. All healthy creatures are content with simple natural foods and sexuality. Healthy people do not need fancy gourmet foods, rich fatty foods, animal foods, luxuries or artificial practices to stimulate their jaded appetite or find pleasure.

3. *Deep, peaceful sleep*: A healthy person falls asleep easily, sleeps without dreams and awakens spontaneously at a predetermined hour, without an alarm clock, and refreshed with 5-8 hours of sleep (less in summer, more in winter).

4. *Good memory*: All learning, growth, and success is based on memory. A healthy person easily recalls past events and experiences as needed. A healthy person's memory improves with age.

5. *Good humor*: Good humor *includes* a cheerful demeanor, deep gratitude, constant enthusiasm, serenity, courage, and love and admiration for all beings and things. Good humor *excludes* greed, hatred, envy, jealousy, frustration, depression, anxiety, nervousness, lust, attachment, brooding, whining or complaining.

6. *Clarity of thought and deed*: A healthy person thinks, judges, speaks and acts with clarity, honesty, precision, and promptness, responding skillfully to all challenges, and establishes order and beauty everywhere under his or her influence.

7. *Honesty*: One strives to live a strong, honest, righteous, virtuous, noble life in alignment with Nature and in search of eternal truth. One denounces degeneracy, dishonesty, immorality and tyranny and promotes health, happiness, virtue and freedom. One feels gratitude for everything, including especially challenges and obstacles.

SICKNESS

Oriental medicine has a preventive perspective, expressed in the following phrase from the *Yellow Emperor's Classic of Internal Medicine*:

> Those who wait to treat disease until it has already arisen are like those who wait until they are thirsty to dig a well, or wait until they are in battle to forge weapons. Are not these actions too late?

Hence, for several thousand years Chinese physicians focused on identifying early signs of imbalance so that they could take actions to avert health disasters by adjusting their own, and their patient's diets and lifestyles. Overt degenerative diseases are always preceded by a long gradual process of apparently minor alterations in health that heralded the oncoming disaster and offered opportunities for self-correction. If you understand why disorder emerges and how it progresses from minor to major, you can interrupt the process using food and lifestyle adjustments, before it become difficult to uproot.

When given excess nutrients in the form of rich foods (especially animal products), the human circulatory system and tissue pathways easily get clogged up. Depending on the amount and duration of the excessive intake of rich food, the body will develop a disorder of adjustment or degeneration.

When acutely exposed to an excess factor, the body will adjust its functions in order to discharge the excess factor(s) and restore homeostasis. For a simple example, if one consumes excess fluids, the body will definitely increase urination and may produce looser stools, and, depending on the climate, more sweat or a runny nose to remove the surplus. Various temporary symptoms such as coughing, fevers, chills, rashes, irritability, excitement, hyperactivity, and such may indicate the body making an adjustment.

When chronically exposed to an excess factor or, less commonly, a deficiency, body systems begin to break down and fluids, cells, tissues, and organs alter in function or structure as a consequence.

In general, as outlined by Michio Kushi,[1] disorder progresses in the following manner:

1. Abnormal discharge and general fatigue
2. Sluggish circulation with aches and pains
3. Blood disorders with chronic discharge
4. Accumulation of excess material in blood and tissues
5. Storage of excess material in tissues and organs
6. Nervous system disorders
7. Spiritual disease

The following provides more detail on these stages:

Stage 1: Fatigue and abnormal discharge: When an individual acutely consumes nutrients in amounts greater than the body can discharge through normal urination, defecation, perspiration, respiration, or physical or mental activity, the overload leads to alterations in function aimed at moving the excess input out of the body, such as: increased defecation, urination, perspiration, or respiration; coughing and sneezing; nausea and vomiting; fidgeting, tapping, muscle twitches, spasms and tension; acute hyperactivity; rapid blinking; irritability, anger, anxiety, excitability, crying, shouting, or screaming.

If an individual recognizes his or her error and adjusts food intake, exercise and rest to allow for recovery of balance between intake and discharge, the body systems will correct itself within a few days. However, if the excess intake continues in spite of the symptoms, the rate of discharge will not keep pace with the rate at which the excess is entering the body. In this case the excess nutrients will begin to cause congestion in the circulatory system, leading to stage 2.

Stage 2: Sluggish circulation: As the rate of intake of excess nutrients from rich foods (particularly animal products, fats, oils, and concentrated sugars) exceeds the body's ability to discharge the excess through the normal channels and the abnormalities that characterize stage 1, the excess nutrients begin accumulating in the blood. This creates thicker, stickier blood that can't properly circulate, nourish, lubricate, or detoxify tissues and organs. The tissues don't get enough oxygen and nutrients, and waste products accumulate faster than they are removed. As the tissues are deprived of oxygen and increasingly loaded with waste products, the individual begins to experience various aches, pains and minor malfunctions such as muscle tension, headaches, menstrual clots and cramps, intermittent numbness, intermittent abdominal discomfort, sleep disturbances, coordination problems, and erratic emotions, mood and attitude.

If the intake of excess nutrients is discontinued at this stage, the body can discharge them and return to healthy function within a few weeks. If the excessive intake continues, the individual will progress to stage 3.

Stage 3: Blood disorders: If one continues to eat excess rich food, the blood becomes progressively saturated with superfluous cholesterol, fat, sugar, amino acids, minerals, and metabolic waste products. This results in temporary or slight but significant changes in blood composition such as anemia, high or low blood sugar, high cholesterol, high triglycerides, and the like.

As the blood becomes more and more saturated with nutriment, blood flow becomes more and more compromised. Impaired circulation to the lungs, large intestine, liver, kidneys, and skin vessels and pores reduces the body's ability to discharge waste products. The increasingly toxic blood, in turn, can't properly nourish, moisten, and detoxify the skin and mucous membranes, which then become more prone to infections. Chronic or recurrent asthma, allergies, and sinus issues may emerge, along with more persistent aches and pains, emotional instability, overly oily or dry skin, acne, and digestive disorders.

When the blood constantly contains excess nutrients (amino acids, fatty acids, cholesterol, etc.), and the immune system is impaired by rising levels of toxic wastes, abnormal growth of rogue cells can occur unchecked, producing first benign tissue overgrowths like skin tags, moles, bunions, and so on. If left unchecked, this process eventually leads to malignant growths.

As the blood becomes more imbalanced, so does the nervous system, resulting in more chronic mental and emotional disorders, such as nervousness, oversensitivity, depression, hyperactivity, confusion, disorientation (loss of purpose), and conflict with family, community and Nature.

The internal build-up of both nutrients and waste products in the blood can cause abnormal sweating, rapid respiration, frequent urination, bad breath, chronic vaginal discharges, and chronic unpleasant body odor.

At this stage, restoration of internal balance will require sticking to a regimen of corrective diet, exercise and rest for at least several weeks and more often several months. It may also be necessary to use additional interventions such as herbal medicines, acupuncture, and body therapies. If nothing is done one will eventually progress to stage 4.

Stage 4: Accumulation of excess: At this stage the blood and tissue levels of water, sugar, fat, cholesterol, amino acids, minerals, and metabolic waste products are chronically elevated and the excess in the blood begins spill over into tissues and organs. The progressive accumulation of excess nutrients, fluids and waste products in the tissues reduces physical mobility, and puts burdens on the internal organs, causing various functional disorders. The now toxic and supersaturated body becomes a fertile ground for infections by viruses, bacteria, and fungi. At this stage, imbalances in the nervous system may produce chronic depression, worry, anger, impatience, frustration, fear, nervousness, timidity, and mental dullness. One may find oneself unable to control one's speech and expressions. Recovery from this stage may require adhering to a therapeutic regimen of diet, exercise, and rest for at least several months.

Stage 5: Storage and organic disorders: At this stage the excess sugar, fat, cholesterol, amino acids, minerals, and/or metabolic waste products have increased in concentration in internal compartments, producing various sediments and supporting abnormal growths and tumors that affect the organic structure of the internal tissues or organs, such as stones, spurs, abnormal tissue growth (e.g. endometriosis), cysts, arteriosclerosis, and, in the most advanced and toxic situations, cancers. It is possible to recover from this stage of imbalance in several months to a year if one adopts a proper program of diet, exercise, and rest.

Stage 6: Nervous system disorders: Since the central nervous system is the information processing and decision-making center for the body, necessary for harmonious function of the various organs and tissues, the body is organized to keep this system from damage for as long as possible. However, like every other tissue of the body, the nerves depend on blood circulation to receive nutrients and oxygen and to remove wastes. If the blood is chronically supersaturated with fats, cholesterol, sugar, and waste products, and blood vessels feeding the nerves become atherosclerotic, the nerves will suffer from chronic malnutrition, toxicity, and oxygen deprivation, resulting in progressive nervous system dysfunction, scarring, and plaque formation. This process results in disorders such as physical paralysis, loss of coordination, suicidal ideation, paranoia, schizophrenia, and violent outbursts, as well as organic diseases such as dementia, Parkinson's disease, and multiple sclerosis. An individual who has reached this stage of imbalance will have to adhere to a therapeutic lifestyle regimen, and get plenty of support from family or friends, for at least 6 months and up to several years, to recover health.

Stage 7: Spiritual disease: At this stage, which one may reach without clearly experiencing all of the previous stages, one refuses to take responsibility for one's own thoughts, words, deeds, and actions. One blames other people, Nature, or God, and refuses to change any habits. Other signs and symptoms of this level of sickness include:

- Self-pity
- Self-centeredness
- Carelessness
- Dishonesty
- Covetousness
- Lack of self-discipline
- Meekness
- Self-indulgence
- Disloyalty
- Disrespectfulness
- Cowardice
- Negligence
- Indolence
- Dependence

- Entitlement
- Spitefulness
- Arrogance

In fact, arrogance – rebellion against Nature, Reality, Truth – is not only the final result but also the first cause of all other diseases and disorders.

This is the deepest level of sickness, for unless one is sick of being sick, one can't become well. On the other hand:

> If one is sick of sickness, then one is not sick.
>
> TAO TE CHING
> CHAPTER 71

LEVELS OF MEDICINE

Oriental medicine has been in development for very likely 5000 years at least. It has traditionally recognized three different grades of medical practice:

The lowest grade of medicine treats only symptoms of disease using natural or artificial drugs and surgical procedures.

The middle grade of medicine identifies and removes the cause of the disorder, through improvement of food intake, physical activity, energy flow, and mental habits and attitudes.

The highest grade of medicine consists of guiding people to an understanding of Natural Law (action and consequences; *karma*) which enables people to reclaim self-respect, self-discipline, and self-governance (sovereignty), so they can elevate their character and way of life.

Oriental medicine also recognizes three grades of physicians:

The lowest grade doctors treat and temporarily relieve symptoms but do not provide guidance to prevention and removal of causes of disease.

The middle grade physicians identify diet and lifestyle causes of disorder and help afflicted individuals change their personal habits.

The highest grade physicians heal disorders of individuals, families, communities and nations through education about Natural Law and Justice and the Way of living harmony with Nature.

NOTES

[1] Adapted from Kushi M, The Book of Macrobiotics (Japan Publications, 1977), pp. 110-12.

4: MACROBIOTIC DIET

Although we *can* eat all types of plant and animal foods, most humans are generally most suited to a predominantly plant-based diet. Christoph Wilhelm Hufeland (1762-1836), the German physician who first used the word "macrobiotics" to describe the art of prolonging life, wrote:

> "In the choice of food one should incline more to vegetables. Flesh has always a greater tendency to putrefaction; and vegetables, on the other hand, to acidity, which corrects putrefaction, our continual and greatest enemy. Besides, animal food is always of a more heating and stimulating nature; whereas vegetables produce cool, mild blood; lessen the internal motion, mental as well as bodily irritability; and powerfully retard vital consumption. Lastly, animal food yields more blood and nourishment; and requires, in order to be beneficial to us, much more labor and bodily motion; and, by the use of it, one also is liable to become plethoric." [1]

Hufeland's traditional Western medicine perspective resonates with traditional Chinese medicine, which prescribes a *qing dan* (light bland) diet composed primarily of whole grains, beans and bean products, vegetables, fruits, nuts and seeds, with animal protein eaten sparingly and not every day. According to Chinese medical principles, grains, beans, vegetables and fruits promote the rising of the clear qi (vitality), while animal foods are rich, heavy, and dense so they tend to weigh down the qi and clog up the fine vessels of the body. Flesh from mammals is more similar to ours than flesh from birds, and flesh from birds is more similar than flesh from fish. Hence mammal's meat is richer than poultry, and poultry is richer than fish.

In addition, Oriental medicine agrees with the traditional Western medical idea, expressed by Hufeland in the above passage, that animal flesh generally has a heating (yang) influence on the body. Consequently, it is easy to ingest an excess of nutrition from animal products – particularly those from mammals – which will burden the digestive process, blood and tissues with excess nutriment and heat, causing one to become, in Hufeland's word, plethoric (overloaded), unless one is engaged in a lot of physical activity and/or inhabiting a cold climate without much shelter or indoor heating.

In Chinese medicine we have a saying: "If flow, no pain; if pain, no flow." In other words, every disease (pain) involves a restriction of blood flow through the painful region. Western medicine agrees that every cell in the body depends on blood circulation for delivery of nutrients and removal of wastes, hence any impairment of blood circulation results in reduced nourishment and increased toxicity of any cell, tissue, or organ affected by the restriction.

Generally, the thicker and stickier the fat and the more nutriment provided by food, the greater its propensity to restrict circulation in the fine arteries of the body, i.e. the more saturated fats like suet, lard, and butter, which are more solid at human body temperature, are more harmful to circulation, whereas the more liquid unsaturated fats like those found in nuts, rapeseed/canola, sesame seed, olives, avocados and fish are neutral or beneficial. Clogging of the vessels from high loads of excess saturated fats and other nutrients can cause digestive issues, fat and phlegm accumulations, and blood stagnation and toxicity, and lead to blood and tissue congestion, stiffness, tension, abnormal sediments, growths and tumors, and edema and heat (inflammation) in affected tissues.

Western science has very well established that diets rich in animal protein, saturated fats, and cholesterol promote increases in blood levels of purines, urea, uric acid, fats and cholesterol, and that this change in blood quality in turn can cause problems like gout and atherosclerosis.[2] Increases in fats, cholesterol, and sugar in the blood make the blood thicker and stickier, which impairs blood flow. Atherosclerosis narrows blood vessels, further impairing blood flow.

Reduced blood flow to the heart causes angina and heart attacks; to the brain and nerves, neural diseases and strokes; to the lower back, back pain;[3] to the genitals, impaired sexual function and fertility such as erectile dysfunction; to the gut, gut diseases like mesenteric ischemia; to the eyes, eye diseases such as "eye stroke"; to the bones, bone diseases; to the kidneys, kidney diseases; and so on. In addition, regular ingestion of large amounts of rich animal products fills our blood with excesses of sulfur-rich amino acids, purines, arachidonic acid, heme iron and other minerals, which in excess are toxic to cells, tissues, and organs. Animal products are also the primary sources of food borne infections (parasites, viruses and bacteria). Consequently a diet excessively rich in animal products can poison the body and cause or promote obesity, cancers, diabetes and its consequences, degenerative joint diseases, auto-immune diseases, and digestive system diseases.[4]

The fact that humans develop atherosclerosis when eating diets rich in animal products proves that we are naturally adapted to plant-based diets, because only animals naturally adapted to plant-based diets can develop atherosclerosis when they regularly eat a diet too rich in animal products.[5,6]

Thus, eating an excess of animal products–particularly those from mammals and especially from animals fattened on grains–promotes the blood and vessel conditions that invite all other degenerative diseases that cause unhappiness and shorten life.

While diets dominated by rich animal products promote disease, diets predominantly composed of whole plant foods – whole grain cereals, legumes, vegetables, seeds, nuts and fruits – prevent and in some cases may reverse disease.[7, 8] Careful scientific research by multiple investigators has demonstrated that if people who have advanced heart disease greatly reduce consumption of land animal flesh, eggs, and milk products to no more than 15% of the diet, the arteries to their hearts will open up and their hearts will heal.[9]

A large body of evidence accumulated over the past 150 years indicates that diets containing a large proportion of land animal protein or more saturated animal fats increase the risk of cardiovascular disease, diabetes, cancer, dementia, auto-immune diseases, osteoporosis, osteoarthritis, allergies, infertility, impotence, back pain, and skin conditions, just to name a few.[10] Additional evidence indicates that diets too rich in land animal protein or fat cause or contribute to many minor afflictions, including acne and other skin issues, constipation, diarrhea, infertility, impotence, menstrual disorders, sensory disturbances, premature aging, depression, and others.

There is no strong evidence that high protein diets improve muscle mass or physical performance, but high intakes of animal protein may contribute to the development of insulin resistance, diabetes, deleterious changes in kidney function, kidney enlargement, renal cell cancer, prostate cancer, kidney stone formation, and metabolic acidosis (which may cause decreased thyroid function). Consequently it is prudent to keep total protein intake to no more than 2 g per kg bodyweight per day.[11]

It has been found that people aged 50-65 who obtained 20% or more of their energy from animal protein had a 75% increase in total mortality, a 4-fold increase in cancer and a 73-fold increase in diabetes mortality during an 18 year observation period.[12] Twenty-percent of kcalories from animal protein equates to 50 g animal protein or about 200 g (7 ounces) of animal flesh per 1000 kcal (14 ounces or nearly a pound of meat per 2000 calories). That's a pretty meaty diet.

In that same study, a "moderate" primarily animal protein intake (10-19% of energy) was associated with a 23-fold increased risk in death from diabetes and a 3-fold increased risk of death from cancer. Plant-based protein was not associated with increased cancer or total mortality. Also, in individuals past the age of 65, higher protein intake was associated with reduced cancer and overall mortality.

Chinese physicians have long noted that peasants generally maintained better health than wealthy people, because they ate simple diets and did plenty of hard work. The famous Chinese doctor Zhu Dan-xi wrote: "Those poor and humble people in the mountains and wilderness know nothing but a bland and homely (diet), but their movements never betray decrepitude and their bodies remain safe and sound (their entire lives)." [13]

This is exemplified by the long-lived Abkhasians of the Caucasus. They ate a predominantly plant-based diet, eating fermented milk products daily, animal flesh only once or twice a week, and only two or three eggs weekly. Among the Abkhasians, "Fat from meat and poultry is not used at all, and butter very seldom. When meat is served, even the smallest pieces of fat are removed, and the people show a great dislike for fatty dishes."[14] Although they consumed fermented (mostly goat) milk products daily, their primarily whole foods plant-based diet provided an average of only 65-73 grams of protein daily (about 15% of energy), an amount easily provided by a strictly whole foods plant based diet and about 50% less than the average in the U.S.A.. Abkhasian centenarians had an average serum cholesterol of only 95 mg/dL,[15] similar to people eating strictly plant-based diets, about half of the average of 192 mg/dL for the U.S. population in 2011-14.[16]

On average, vegetarian Seventh Day Adventists have one of the longest healthy life spans of any well-described natural population in the modern world.[17] They live an average of almost 10 years longer than non-vegetarian non-Adventist Americans, and without disability. Their main advantage? A very low risk of heart and cardiovascular disease deaths.[18] Among Adventist men, total mortality rates are lowest and similar for either vegans or pesco-vegetarians (who may consume dairy products and eggs as well as fish at least once a month), but among Adventist women, total mortality rates are lowest among pesco-vegetarians and semi-vegetarians (who consumed nonfish meats 1 time/mo or more and all animal flesh including fish 1 time/mo or more but no more than 1 time/wk).[19]

Japanese consistently rank at the top or within the top 2 or 3 nations for life expectancy. Within Japan and possibly the world, the Okinawans have the greatest life expectancy, primarily because they avoid or delay major age-related diseases.[20] Okinawa apparently produces more centenarians than any other region of the contemporary world, and almost two-thirds of Okinawans function independently at age 97.

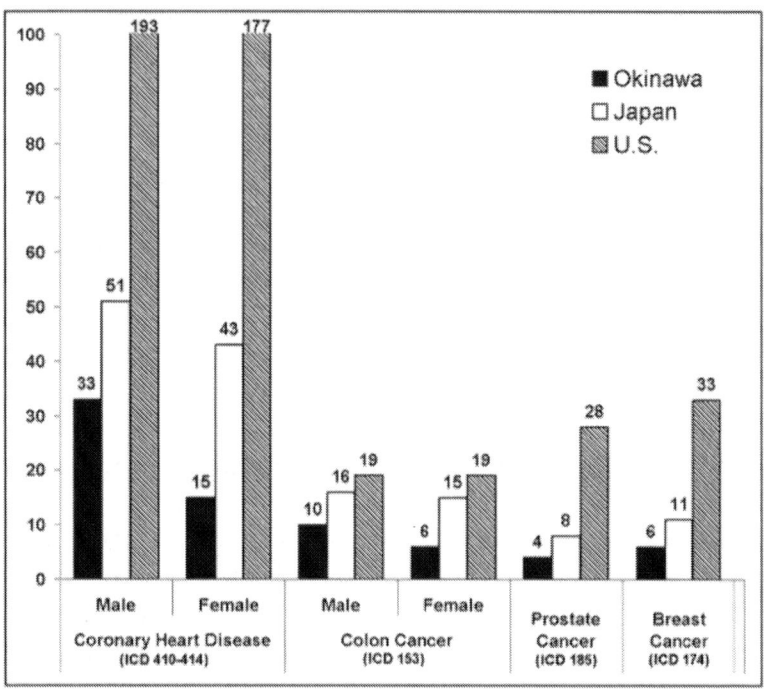

Figure 6.1: Mortality rates from coronary heart disease and cancers in Okinawans, Japanese, and Americans.[30]

In 1949 the traditional Okinawan diet consisted primarily (98%) of whole plant foods including sweet potatoes (their staple), legumes (mostly tofu), land and sea vegetables (typically stir-fried in oil), local fruits, tea, and herbs; only about 1% of calories came from animals, mostly fish. Since then prosperity has enabled them to increase their intake of animal food, but Okinawans still get about 85% of their energy from whole plant foods. Their diet and lifestyle largely liberates them from heart disease and cancers common in nations where typical diets are rich in land animal products, such as the U.S.A. (Figure 3.1).

In contemporary South Korea, centenarians consume a primarily plant-based diet that is by weight 87% plant foods (only about 3.5 ounces of total animal products daily, primarily fish).[21]

Nordic peoples who adhere more closely to a healthy Nordic food diet consisting of locally sourced wild fish, cabbages, rye bread, oatmeal, apples and pears, local berries, and root vegetables have a lower annual rate of deaths from all causes compared to those who eat more land animal products and saturated fats.[22, 23]

In a comparison of five long-lived populations (Japanese in Japan, Swedes in Sweden, Anglo-Celtic in Australia, Greeks in Australia and Greece), researchers found that the three dietary factors most associated with protection against premature death from degenerative disease were 1) high ratio of monounsaturated to saturated fats, 2) high intake of legumes, and 3) regular consumption of fish.[24] Intakes of cereals, fruits, vegetables, and nuts were neutral, and meat, dairy, and alcohol intake were found potentially harmful.

Completely vegetarian diets are not likely suitable for all people. Genetic research indicates that about 83% Europeans and 70% of East Asians probably have a dietary requirement for the omega-3 fat DHA due to a limited ability to produce it from precursors supplied by plants.[25]

So, as a general rule, all other factors being equal, it appears that *eating excess land animal protein and saturated fats promotes premature disability and disease*, but, *wild fish may in limited amounts be beneficial to health and longevity.*

In summary, humans appear best adapted to a varied, primarily plant-based diet supplemented regularly with fish, or with meat or eggs from wild or pastured birds, and perhaps occasionally with meat or milk from wild or pastured animals.

Ecological Cost of Eating Animal Foods

More than 2000 years ago, in Plato's REPUBLIC, Socrates pointed out that a community that depends on raising animals for food will generally require more land and other resources than one that depends on a vegetarian diet. This remains generally true today. Consider these facts[26]:

Soil Depletion
- U.S. livestock consume five times as much grain as is consumed directly by the entire U.S. human population.
- On average, it takes 6 kg of plant protein to produce just 1 kg of animal protein.
- More than 302 million hectares of land are devoted to feeding the U.S. livestock population – 272 million hectares in pasture and about 30 million hectares for producing feed grains.
- Ninety percent of U.S. croplands are losing soil at an average of 13 times the sustainable rate due to wind and water erosion caused by intensive cropping to produce livestock feed grains. Some of the richest farming areas are being depleted even faster; Iowa loses topsoil at 30 times the rate of soil formation, and has lost one-half of its topsoil in just 150 years of farming.
- Erosion of pasture lands amounts to 6 tons per hectare per year on average, but may exceed 100 tons on severely overgrazed pastures, and 54 percent of U.S. pastureland is overgrazed.

Water Usage
- Production of one gram of protein from milk, eggs, or chicken flesh uses 50% more water than production of a gram of protein from pulses (beans, peas, lentils). For beef, the water cost per gram of protein is 6 times larger than for pulses.[27]

Air and Water Pollution
- Livestock operations produce more than 335 million tons of manure annually.[28]
- Concentrated animal manure from modern animal feeding operations pollutes fresh water and air. Animal waste has contaminated drinking water supplies, rivers, streams, and the oceans.[29]

Fossil Fuel Demands
- On average, it takes 28 kilocalories (kcal) of fossil fuel input to produce 1 kcal of animal protein for human consumption. In contrast, it takes only 3.3 kcal of fossil fuel to produce 1 kcal of grain protein for human consumption.
- Some 17 percent of the total energy the U.S. spends goes to support production of meat for human consumption.[30]
- Production of the typical U.S. diet requires twice as much fossil fuel as a lacto-ovo-vegetarian diet, and three times as much fuel as a vegan diet.[31]

Ocean Depletion
- Fifty-three percent of ocean fisheries are at or close to their maximum sustainable productions, with no room for further expansion, and 32 percent are either overexploited (28 percent), depleted (3 percent), or recovering from depletion (1 percent).[32]
- For every pound of ocean fish caught for human consumption, up to 5 pounds of unintended marine species are caught and discarded as by-kill.[33]
- Human-caused erosion of ocean biodiversity appears to be accelerating world-wide, and it is predicted that all fish stocks currently fished will collapse in 2048.[34]
- Dead zones in the oceans are primarily caused by nitrogen and phosphorous runoff from agriculture.[35]

Deforestation
- Cattle ranching is the primary driver of deforestation in the Brazilian Amazon.[36]

Most of these problems are primarily caused by government subsidies. U.S. politicians provide the animal food industry with hundreds of billions of dollars annually in subsidies and favors that supply cheap or free fuel, water or land to farmers and ranchers, encourage overgrazing on public lands and overproduction of crops fed to animals, and protect confined animal feeding operations (CAFOs) from the costs of proper disposal of animal wastes.[37] Legislators have also instituted laws against public criticism of products and practices of the livestock industry (i.e. anti-free speech laws: ag-gag and food libel laws), and given the industry protection from legal responsibility for pollution of waterways. U.S. politicians also provide more than $700 million annually in subsidies to the fishing industry, which encourages overfishing and protects the industry from costs that would drive up the market price of fish.[38] Stopping the subsidies would stop the waste.

Most Americans have an animal protein intake alone that is double basic requirements, disregarding plant protein. If the U.S. livestock industry only raised animals on pasture, it would still produce enough animal products to give every U.S. citizen the amount of animal protein found in about 4 ounces of lean meat daily[39] (about half of protein needs) and these animal products would have nutritional profiles more like wild fish, lower in total and saturated fats and richer in essential omega-3 fats. Eating less conventional animal products and more plant protein reduces our demands on natural resources. Avoiding or minimizing beef consumption reduces the environmental costs of diet most effectively.[40]

Universal Macrobiotic Diet Recommendations

- Study and implement the dietary practices of your healthy preindustrial and preagricultural ancestors.
- Make your diet as plant-based as practical for your heritage and location.
- Choose foods adapted to your bioregion and the current season. Avoid imported foods.
- Choose the highest quality, most naturally produced foods your budget will allow.
- Choose foods produced by permaculture methods whenever possible.
- Grow your own foods whenever possible.
- Choose foods appropriate for your personal constitution and condition.
- If eating animal foods, generally give first preference to wild fish, and otherwise to locally sourced products from wild game or animals exclusively fed their natural, species-appropriate diets. Whenever practical, choose fish over poultry, and poultry over mammal's meat. However, adjust this to your local food resources. Avoid mass produced commercial animal products from animals fed artificial (usually grain-based) diets, chemicals and drugs.
- If you choose not to eat wild game or fish at least once weekly, you must take a B12 supplement (see B12 section below).
- If you do not consume at least 200 g weekly of fatty fish, you must take a minimum of 250 mg/day of algal-source (vegan) DHA.[41]
- Seek a balance of the five flavors–salty, sweet, sour, bitter, and pungent–and of *yin* and *yang* influences in harmony with bioregion, climate, season, and individual needs.

Specific Temperate Zone Guidelines

- Main foods at most meals:
  - Whole cereal grains
  - Legumes (beans, peas, lentils)
  - Starchy roots or tubers
  - Starchy nuts (e.g. acorns, chestnuts)
- Land and sea vegetables, fungi, fruits, seeds, nuts, animal products, herbs and seasonings compose the remainder of the diet.
- Generally limit lean wild or pastured animal products to no more than 15% of energy intake, which amounts to about 100 g (3.5 ounces) lean animal flesh per 1000 kcal in the diet (see Animal Product section below).

Whole Cereal Grains and Cereal Grain Products

- Whole cereal grains include brown rice, whole wheat, whole corn, barley, oats, sorghum, spelt, millet, teff, rye, wild rice, triticale and others. Amaranth, buckwheat, and quinoa are pseudocereals.
- At least 95% of your cereal grain intake should consist of whole cereal grains.
- Favor the staple cereals of your ancestors.
- You may use locally produced starchy roots or tubers as alternatives to cereals.
- You may regularly, even daily include whole grain noodles, pasta, and breads.
- Moist, boiled and steamed preparations are preferable to dry, baked preparations (e.g. steamed bread instead of baked bread).
- Choose grains grown with permaculture or natural farming methods whenever possible.

Legumes and Plant-Based Meats

- Generally, legumes are more nourishing for humans and the soil than cereals. In some studies, legume intake is more strongly associated with longevity than any other food.[42]
- Smaller beans like adzuki, mung, chickpeas (garbanzos), small black beans, and various lentils and peas are easiest to digest hence best for regular use.
- Emphasize consuming legumes that your ancestors consumed.
- If not eating animal products, include *at least* 3 servings of legumes, legume products, or plant-based meats in the general daily diet. A serving provides 7 g protein (similar to 1 ounce of animal flesh) and consists of
  - 1/2 cup of whole cooked legumes
  - 1/4 block of tofu
  - 1.5 ounce of tempeh
  - 8 ounces of unsweetened soy milk
  - 1.25 ounce of plant-based meat such as seitan/wheat meat or commercial vegan meat alternates.
- Generally whole legumes or tempeh should constitute at least half of your legume intake.

Seeds

- Generally include about 1-2 ounces of oil-rich whole seeds in your daily diet. Amount may vary according to individual condition, activity level, season, time, and place.
- Oily skin or acne may indicate an excess of oil in your diet. Cold weather, dry climates, and high levels of physical activity may increase one's need for oils from seeds or nuts. Cravings for animal fats, body dryness, intolerance of cold weather, and swings in energy levels may indicate a need for more seeds or nuts in the diet.

- Beneficial seeds include sesame, sunflower, pumpkin, hemp, chia, and flax.

Vegetables

- Make fresh vegetables comprise roughly 25-30% of total food volume *on average*. These serve as your primary source of vitamins A and C and some minerals.
- Aim to eat at least 5 different vegetables every day, including as a general baseline
    - 1 cup of dark green leafy vegetables (e.g. kale, bok choy)
    - 1/2-1 cup of root vegetables (e.g. carrots, daikon)
    - 1/2-1 cup of round vegetables (e.g. onions, cabbage, winter squash)
    - 5-10 grams of sea vegetables
- Whenever possible choose locally grown vegetables.
- Wash produce to remove any pesticides, or purchase pesticide-free produce if your budget allows.
- Raw vegetables have limited nutritional value because humans lack the enzymes to digest cellulose and therefore have limited access to the nutrients in raw vegetables.
- Consume most of your vegetables properly cooked in various styles such as lightly steamed or boiled, sautéed in broth or with a *very* small amount of unrefined, cold pressed oil (see guidelines below), etc..
- Fermentation (natural pickling) improves the nutritional value of raw plant foods. You may consume a very small volume of naturally fermented vegetables daily.
- Onions, leeks or garlic are odorous and may arouse passions such as anger and lust. On the other hand, allium family vegetables have strong health-promotion properties. Exercise your own discretion in their use.
- Land vegetables to use regularly include, but are not limited to: green cabbage, kale, broccoli, cauliflower,

celery, collards, pumpkin, watercress, parsley, Chinese cabbage, bok choy, dandelion, mustard greens, daikon greens, scallion, onions, sweet peppers, daikon radish, turnips, burdock, beets, carrots, sweet potatoes, and winter squash such as kabocha, butternut, buttercup, and acorn squash.
- Land vegetables to use cooked or occasionally raw in hot seasons or climates include cucumber, celery, lettuce, spinach, tomato, summer squash, and herbs such as dill and chives.
- Limit the nightshade family vegetables – potatoes, tomatoes, and eggplant–to occasional use.
- Have a small serving of sea vegetables daily, choosing from kelp/kombu, alaria, nori, dulse, sea palm, ocean ribbons, wakame, arame, hijiki, and others.
- Consume fungi (various mushrooms and yeasts) on a regular basis, including especially shiitake mushrooms and nutritional yeast.

Nuts

- Up until recent times, nut consumption was very limited by the difficulty of extracting the meats from shells.
- Some people find that nuts are difficult to digest, and a common cause of allergies and skin rashes.
- Limit nut intake to no more than one ounce daily.
- Prefer nuts grown in a bioregion similar to your own habitat. Recommended nuts for people inhabiting temperate regions include almonds, pecans, hazelnuts/filberts, pine nuts, and walnuts, or other locally available nuts.

Fruits

- Most fruits have more yin characteristics: sweet and sour flavor and a cool or cold thermal effect. With a few

- exceptions, they generally clear heat, moisten dryness, dissolve phlegm, produce body fluids, and increase urination.
- In Chinese medicine, some fruits, including jujube dates (hong zao) and lycium berries (gou qi zi), are highly regarded for their specific health and longevity benefits.
- Consumption of at least two servings of fruit daily has been associated with a lower risk of all cause mortality.[43]
- In general, palm dates, jujube dates, and various berries, including grapes, are highly beneficial in small amounts.
- Consume fresh or dried fruits daily, according to climate, season and individual condition.
- Generally choose locally grown fruits or those grown in a bioregion and climate similar to that which you inhabit. Avoid or minimize fruits imported from bioregions and climates very different from the one you inhabit.
- Use organic fruit if your budget permits but if not, eat the best quality locally grown fruits you can find.

Animal Products

- If you choose not to eat animal products, you must take supplements of vitamin B12 and omega-3 DHA.
- If you choose to eat animal products, use only the best quality available in small amounts as supplementary foods. High quality animal products include:
  - Wild fish and game meats
  - Products from exclusively pasture-fed animals
  - Products from animals raised as parts of sustainable aquaculture or permaculture systems
- Avoid all commercial animal products since they come from animals that have been abused, fed concentrated feed that makes them artificially fat, or given hormones or drugs. Flesh, eggs, and milk from such animals are nutritionally harmful.

- Avoid concentrated animal fats, including butter and fat from meat or poultry such as lard, suet or others.
- Fish intake is the second most important dietary predictor of longevity (behind legumes).[44]
  - The optimal seafood consumption to balance nutrient benefits with risks (mercury, arsenic, etc.) appears to be about 200 g of fatty fish (swordfish, herring, halibut, salmon, mackerel, sardines) and 50 g lean fish per week.[45] Limit lean wild or pastured animal products to no more than 15% of your daily energy intake.
- Current evidence suggests it is prudent to avoid consuming more than 2 g total protein per kg per day.[46] It would also be prudent to obtain at least half of one's total protein from plant foods. This would limit animal protein intake to half of total protein, as shown in Table 6.1. This corresponds to limiting animal flesh to no more than 15% of total caloric intake (Table 6.2).

Table 6.1: Suggested upper limit for daily animal protein (PRO) intake.			
Body mass kg (lbs)	Max. total PRO g	Max. animal PRO g	Max. animal flesh intake g (oz)
45 (100)	90	45	180 (6)
57 (125)	114	57	240 (8)
68 (150)	136	68	290 (10)
78 (175)	156	78	334 (11)
90 (200)	180	90	386 (13)

- Since lean game, wild fish, or pastured animal flesh generally provide about 1.6 kcal per gram (~45 kcal per ounce), that allows about 100 g (3.5 oz.) of lean animal flesh per 1000 calories consumed (Table 6.2).
- Generally, people who inhabit more northern climates must eat more animal foods due to lesser plant food availability.

Table 6.2: General Upper Limits (UL) for Animal Product Consumption Based on Energy Intake[1]		
Daily Energy Intake (kcalories)	**Animal Product UL (kcalories)**	**Animal Product UL (g/oz lean MFP)[2]**
1500	225	140 g (5 ounces)
2000	300	190 g (7 ounces)
2500	375	235 g (8 ounces)
3000	400	250 g (9 ounces)
3500	525	330 g (12 ounces)

1. Defining upper limit as 15% of calories. 2. Consume only wild caught fish, wild game, or meat from pastured animals fed only the types of foods they would consume in the wild.

Salt

- Salt tolerance or requirements are determined by ancestry.
  - Europeans and Asians generally have a high tolerance for dietary salt, and may have a requirement for it, inherited from ancestors who had to use salt to preserve foods for long winters.

- People of African descent are genetically more likely to be salt sensitive hypertensives[47] because their ancestors did not need to use salt for food preservation.
- Among Europeans, sodium intake below 3 g per day has been associated with higher mortality from cardiovascular disease.[48]
- People who eat animal products have less need for dietary salt compared to those who limit animal products, because animal flesh, eggs, and salt are rich in sodium.
- Some salt is very important for sustaining health on a highly plant-based or vegan diet, as it is the main source of both sodium and chloride (needed for stomach acid production), both poorly supplied by most edible plants.
- Inadequate salt intake will result in loss of appetite, poor digestion, low energy, and lack of mental acuity.
- Research suggests that at least for Europeans and Asians the sweet spot for *sodium* intake lies in the range of 3 to 7 g per day, which equates to 1.5 to 3 level domestic teaspoons daily of salt.[49, 50]
- Use unrefined sea salt and naturally fermented soy products including miso and soy sauce daily in cooking but not at the table (table use typically leads to overuse).
- For a salty table condiment, grind one part roasted sea salt with 8-16 parts roasted sesame seeds (sesame salt: Japanese *gomashio*).

Vegetable Oils

- Vegetable oils are highly processed, highly concentrated fats, with a high propensity to become body fat and have toxic effects.
- Whole seeds and nuts are more beneficial than extracted oils. To reduce body fat or improve health limit or avoid extracted oils in the daily diet.

- Healthy people can generally consume about 1 teaspoon of oil per thousand calories consumed, for the typical person, 2-3 tsp. per day, which amounts to only about 5% of total caloric intake. Your needs may vary.
- A high intake of monounsaturated fat coupled with a low intake of saturated fat is protective against premature death.[51] Oils rich in monounsaturated fat include sesame, rapeseed/canola, and olive.
- Use oils that were consumed by your ancestors prior to modernization and avoid oils not used by your ancestors.
- Use oils that can be or are produced in a bioregion similar to the one you inhabit, and avoid oils from dissimilar regions. For example
    - Southern temperate regions: olive or sesame oils
    - Northern temperate regions: rapeseed/canola oil
    - Tropical regions: palm or coconut oil

Vitamin B-12

- Modern water treatment, agricultural methods, and hygiene practices have reduced the availability of vitamin B-12 in water, vegetal foods, and the general environment.
- "Vitamin B-12 deficiency and depletion are common in wealthier countries, particularly among the elderly, and are most prevalent in poorer populations around the world."[52]
- "Contrary to popular belief, not only strict vegetarians (vegans) are at high risk of vitamin B-12 deficiency, and there is strong evidence that status reflects usual intake across a wide range."[53]
- Humans have difficulty absorbing B-12 from animal-flesh foods, especially as we age.[54]
- Everyone who lives in an urban environment should use foods fortified with vitamin B-12 or take a vitamin B-12

supplement on a regular basis, unless you are consuming traditionally fermented foods with proven B12 content.
- Do not rely on commercially available fermented foods such as pickles, miso or tempeh for B-12 because modern hygienic production methods do not reliably provide B-12, unlike traditional methods.
- Do not rely on algae like spirulina or chlorella for B-12 because at this point in time the bulk of research shows these do not provide active B-12, only an inactive analogue.

Sweet Flavor

- Focus on including plenty of the sweet flavor at meals from whole grains or sweet vegetables including winter squash, carrots, onions, and cabbages properly prepared with sufficient salt (see the Recipe section).
- Use locally produced sweeteners that were used by your ancestors only occasionally (generally not more than a few times weekly) in small amounts, for special occasions or medicine.
  - Temperate region: honey, maple syrup, temperate fruit concentrates and syrups
- Honeys have antibacterial properties and are "very effective wound treatments." [55]
- Europeans and Asians should avoid tropical origin sweeteners including cane sugar and agave.

Sour Flavor

- For a sour taste use umeboshi (pickled plums); vinegar-free naturally fermented vegetable pickles; small amounts of naturally processed vinegars including brown rice vinegar, umeboshi vinegar, apple cider vinegar, or red wine vinegar; or lemon, lime, or orange juice.

Spicy Flavor

- For a pungent flavor in meals, incorporate grated radishes or chopped fresh scallions, or use fresh ginger or various fresh or dried herbs and spices in cooking.
  - You can prepare just about any ethnic food in a macrobiotic style, using garlic and spices skillfully and with restraint.
  - Strong spices and garlic generally balance very heavy, greasy foods and counteract toxins provided by animal flesh, eggs, and dairy products.
  - Eating very spicy food has a dispersing and draining effect that demands counterbalance with heavy, rich, greasy, or animal-based foods. Hence, eating very spicy food can cause cravings for or attraction to heavy, rich, or greasy foods.
  - Keep in mind that if you start to feel light headed, spacey, depleted, or have cravings for fats, oils, or animal products, you may need to cut back on garlic or spices.

Sun Exposure

- Early morning sun exposure is highly recommended and practically essential for maintaining proper hormonal balance and sleep quality. Aim to regularly get at least 15 minutes of natural day light in the dawn hour.
- You need regular unprotected sun exposure to obtain adequate vitamin D. Aim to spend at least 60 minutes out doors each week, during a time when the local UV index is between 2 and 4, preferably split into at least three sessions.

Water and Beverages

- Use clean spring, well, or filtered water for all cooking and drinking. For water filtration I recommend the Multipure drinking water systems; for more information about these systems go to http://www.multipureusa.com/dmatesz/index2.html.
- Drink adequate liquids according to thirst. Do not drink if not thirsty. Generally, you will drink less on a plant-based diet compared to an animal-based diet due to the large amount of fluid provided by plant foods.
- If you need to urinate more than six times in a day, or need to urinate at night, you may be taking too much fluid.
- Do not drink cold beverages with meals as this can impair enzyme-action and digestion.
- Use teas brewed from locally grown plants; avoid beverages made from imported plants
- Substitute roasted grain or root beverages such as roasted barley, dandelion, or chicory, alone or in combination for the coffee flavor.
- Some recommended beverages include: Kukicha twig tea, roasted grain coffee, roasted dandelion tea, roasted chicory tea, roasted barley tea, and local herbal teas.

Food Preparation Suggestions

- If possible, cook on a gas or wood stove, which improves the flavor and quality of the food. If possible, avoid using electric cooking devices as much as practical and upgrade to gas or wood; however, if all you have access to is an electric appliance, don't fret about it; it is more important to eat home-cooked food at regular meal times than to have the food cooked over a live flame. Most importantly, avoid microwave ovens.

- Use earthenware, cast iron, or stainless steel cookware and avoid aluminum or Teflon-coated pots.
- Treat cooking and food preparation as a meditation and opportunity to express your love and care for yourself and others.

Additional Diet Suggestions

- *Eat regular meals*, i.e. at consistent times from day to day. Frequent shifting of mealtimes can contribute to metabolic disorders. Eating regular meals will result in regulation of blood sugar, energy levels, bowel movements, emotions, menstrual cycles, and sleep cycles. In case of any disorder the most important step to restoring order consists of establishing regular meals. Morning and noon are the best meal times.
- Eat food warm or at room temperature, generally avoid cold or frozen foods, as these impair gut and enzyme function.
- Eat only when relaxed; do not eat when emotional.
- During meals, sit with a good posture and take a moment to express gratitude for the food.
- Do not engage in demanding or distracting activities while eating, but put your attention on the food, proper chewing, and the people with whom you share the meal.
- Chew your food thoroughly to mix with saliva and ensure good digestion and assimilation.
- Eat to the point of satisfaction, in balance with your food requirements.

NOTES

[1] Hufeland CW. *Art of Prolonging Life*, ed. by Erasmus Wilson, F.R.S. (Boston: Ticknor, Reed, and Fields, 1854).

[2] Roberts WC. Twenty questions on atherosclerosis. *Proceedings (Baylor University Medical Center)*. 2000;13(2):139-143.
<http://www.ncbi.nlm.nih.gov/pmc/articles/PMC1312295/>

[3] Kauppila LI. Atherosclerosis and disc degeneration/low-back pain--a systematic review. Eur J Vasc Endovasc Surg. 2009 Jun;37(6):661-70.
<http://www.ncbi.nlm.nih.gov/pubmed/19328027>

[4] McDougall JA, *The Starch Solution* (Rodale, 2012).

[5] Roberts WC, op. cit..

[6] Moghadasian MH. Experimental atherosclerosis: A historical overview. Life Sciences 70 (2002) 855–865.

[7] Ibid.

[8] Campbell TC, *Whole* (BenBella Books, 2014).

[9] Campbell TC, *The China Study* (Benbella Books, 2004), pp. 117-130.

[10] Campbell TC, *The China Study* (Benbella Books, 2004).

[11] Metges CC and Barth CA, "Metabolic Consequences of a High Dietary Protein Intake in Adulthood: Assessment of the Available Evidence," J Nutr 2016 Oct;146(10):886-889.
<http://jn.nutrition.org/content/130/4/886.full>

[12] Levine, Morgan E. et al. "Low Protein Intake Is Associated with a Major Reduction in IGF-1, Cancer, and Overall Mortality in the 65 and Younger but Not Older Population." *Cell metabolism* 19.3 (2014): 407–417. *PMC*. Web. 3 Nov. 2016.
<https://www.ncbi.nlm.nih.gov/pmc/articles/PMC3988204/>

[13] Flaws B, *The Book of Jook* (Blue Poppy Enterprises, Inc., 1995), p. 18.

[14] Benet S, *Abkhasians: The Long-Living People of the Caucasus* (Holt, Rinehart and Winston, 1974), p. 25.

[15] Ibid., pp. 21-27.

[16] CDC, National Center for Health Statistics, Cholesterol; dated July 15, 2016. <http://www.cdc.gov/nchs/fastats/cholesterol.htm>

[17] Fraser GE, Shavlik DJ. Ten Years of Life: Is It a Matter of Choice? *Arch Intern Med*. 2001;161(13):1645-1652. doi:10.1001/archinte.161.13.1645. <http://archinte.jamanetwork.com/article.aspx?articleid=648593>

[18] Orlich MJ, Singh PN, Sabaté J, et al. Vegetarian Dietary Patterns and Mortality in Adventist Health Study 2. *JAMA internal medicine*. 2013;173(13):1230-1238. doi:10.1001/jamainternmed.2013.6473. <http://www.ncbi.nlm.nih.gov/pmc/articles/PMC4191896/>

[19] Ibid.

[20] Willcox DC, Willcox BJ, Todoriki H, Suzuki M. The Okinawan Diet: Health Implications of a Low-Calorie, Nutrient-Dense, Antioxidant-Rich Dietary Patter Low in Glycemic Load. J Am Coll Nutr 2009;28(4):500S-516S.

[21] Chung Shil Kwak, Mee Sook Lee, Se In Oh, and Sang Chul Park, "Discovery of Novel Sources of Vitamin B12 in Traditional Korean Foods from Nutritional Surveys of Centenarians," Current Gerontology and Geriatrics Research, vol. 2010, Article ID 374897, 11 pages, 2010. doi:10.1155/2010/374897

[22] Olsen A, Egeberg R, Halkjær J, et al.. Healthy aspects of the Nordic diet are related to lower total mortality. J Nutr. 2011 Apr 1;141(4):639-44. <http://jn.nutrition.org/content/141/4/639.long>

[23] Roswall N, Sandin S, Löf M, et al.. Adherence to the healthy Nordic food index and total and cause-specific mortality among Swedish women. Eur J Epidemiol. 2015 Jun;30(6):509-17.

[24] Darmadi-Blackberry I, Wahlqvist ML, Kouris-Blazos A, Steen B, Lukito W, Horie Y, Horie K. Legumes: the most important dietary predictor of survival in older people of different ethnicities. Asia Pac J Clin Nutr. 2004;13(2):217-20. PubMed PMID: 15228991. p. 219.
http://apjcn.nhri.org.tw/server/APJCN/13/2/217.pdf

[25] Kothapalli KSD, Gadgil MS, Carlson SE, et. al., "Positive selection on a regulatory insertion-deletion polymorphism in FADS2 influences apparent endogenous synthesis of arachidonic acid," Mol Biol Evol 2016 March 29; doi: 10.1093/molbev/msw049.
<http://mbe.oxfordjournals.org/content/early/2016/03/09/molbev.msw049.full.pdf+html>

[26] Unless otherwise noted, this data comes from: Pimental D. Livestock Production: Energy Inputs and the Environment. Cornell Chronicle 7 Aug 1997.
<http://www.news.cornell.edu/stories/1997/08/us-could-feed-800-million-people-grain-livestock-eat>

[27] Mekonnen MM, Hoekstra AY. A Global Assessment of the Water Footprint of Farm Animal Products. Ecosystems (2012);15:401-15.
<http://temp.waterfootprint.org/Reports/Mekonnen-Hoekstra-2012-WaterFootprintFarmAnimalProducts.pdf>

[28] USDA ARS. FY-2005 Annual Report Manure and Byproduct Utilization; National Program 206.
<http://www.ars.usda.gov/research/programs/programs.htm?np_code=206&docid=13337>

[29] EPA. Animal Waste. What's the Problem?
<http://www3.epa.gov/region9/animalwaste/problem.html>

[30] Whitney EN, Rolfes SR. Understanding Nutrition, 6th Edition. West Publishing, 1993. 656.

[31] Ibid. 657.

[32] FAO. World Review of Fisheries and Aquaculture. The State of World Fisheries and Aquaculture 2010. 8.
<http://www.fao.org/docrep/013/i1820e/i1820e01.pdf>

[33] Cluca I. A Study of the Options for the Utilization of Bycatch and Discards from Marine Capture Fisheries. FAO Fisheries Circular No 928.
<http://www.fao.org/docrep/w6602e/w6602e00.HTM>

[34] Worm B, Barbier EB, Beaumont N, et al. Impacts of Biodiversity Loss on Ocean Ecosystem Services. Science 3 Nov 2006;314:787.
<http://www.sciencemag.org/content/314/5800/787.full.pdf>

[35] What Causes Ocean "Dead Zones"? Scientific American 25 Sept 2012.
<http://www.scientificamerican.com/article/ocean-dead-zones/>

[36] Margulis S. Causes of deforestation of the Brazilian Amazon. World Bank, 2004.
<http://www-wds.worldbank.org/servlet/WDSContentServer/WDSP/IB/2004/02/02/000090341_20040202130625/Rendered/PDF/277150PAPER0wbwp0no1022.pdf>

[37] PCRM. Government Support for Unhealthful Foods.
<http://www.pcrm.org/health/reports/agriculture-and-health-policies-unhealthful-foods>

[38] Sharp, R. and U.R. Sumaila. 2009. Quantification of U.S. Marine Fisheries Subsidies. North American Journal of Fisheries Management 29(1): 18-32.
<http://www.lenfestocean.org/~/media/legacy/lenfest/pdfs/sharp_sumaila_2009.pdf?la=en>

[39] Pimental D, op. cit.

[40] Eshel, Gidon et al. "Land, Irrigation Water, Greenhouse Gas, and Reactive Nitrogen Burdens of Meat, Eggs, and Dairy Production in the United States." *Proceedings of the National Academy of Sciences of the United States of America* 111.33 (2014): 11996–12001. *PMC*. Web. 14 Nov. 2016. <https://www.ncbi.nlm.nih.gov/pmc/articles/PMC4143028/>

[41] Sarter B, Kelsey KS, Schwartz TA, et al., "Blood docosahexaenoic acid and eicosapentaenoic acid in vegans: Associations with age and gender and effects of an algal-derived omega-3 fatty acid supplement," Clinical Nutrition 2015;34:212-218.
<http://www.clinicalnutritionjournal.com/article/S0261-5614(14)00076-4/pdf>

[42] Darmadi-Blackberry I, Wahlqvist ML, Kouris-Blazos A, Steen B, Lukito W, Horie Y, Horie K. Legumes: the most important dietary predictor of survival in older people of different ethnicities. Asia Pac J Clin Nutr. 2004;13(2):217-20. PubMed PMID: 15228991.
http://apjcn.nhri.org.tw/server/APJCN/13/2/217.pdf

[43] Wang X, Ouyang Y, Liu J, et al. Fruit and vegetable consumption and mortality from all causes, cardiovascular disease, and cancer: systematic review and dose-response meta-analysis of prospective cohort studies. *The BMJ*. 2014;349:g4490. doi:10.1136/bmj.g4490.
<http://www.ncbi.nlm.nih.gov/pmc/articles/PMC4115152/>

[44] See note 26.

[45] Sirot, V., Leblanc, J.-C. and Margaritis, I. (2011) 'A risk–benefit analysis approach to seafood intake to determine optimal consumption', *British Journal of Nutrition*, 107(12), pp. 1812–1822.

[46] Metges CC and Barth CA, "Metabolic Consequences of a High Dietary Protein Intake in Adulthood: Assessment of the Available Evidence," J Nutr 2016 Oct;146(10):886-889.
<http://jn.nutrition.org/content/130/4/886.full>

[47] American Heart Association. "Hold The Salt: Gene May Explain African Americans' Extra Sensitivity To Salt, Leading To High Blood Pressure." ScienceDaily. ScienceDaily, 26 March 1999.
<www.sciencedaily.com/releases/1999/03/990326061953.htm>.

[48] Stolarz-Skrzypek K, Kuznetsova T, Thijs L, et al. Fatal and Nonfatal Outcomes, Incidence of Hypertension, and Blood Pressure Changes in Relation to Urinary Sodium Excretion. *JAMA*. 2011;305(17):1777-1785.
<http://jama.jamanetwork.com/article.aspx?articleid=899663>

[49] O'Donnell MJ, Yusuf S, Mente A, et al. Urinary Sodium and Potassium Excretion and Risk of Cardiovascular Events. *JAMA*. 2011;306(20):2229-2238.
<http://jama.jamanetwork.com/article.aspx?articleid=1105553>

[50] McMaster University. "Low-salt diets may not be beneficial for all, study suggests: Salt reduction only important in some people with high blood pressure." ScienceDaily. ScienceDaily, 21 May 2016.
<www.sciencedaily.com/releases/2016/05/160521071410.htm>

[51] See note 26.

[52] Allen LH. How common is vitamin B-12 deficiency? Am J Clin Nutr 2009 Feb; 89(2):6935-6965. Accessed on 7/18/16 at <http://ajcn.nutrition.org/content/89/2/693S.long>

[53] Ibid.

[54] Ibid.

[55] Carter, Dee A. et al. "Therapeutic Manuka Honey: No Longer So Alternative." *Frontiers in Microbiology* 7 (2016): 569. *PMC*. Web. 22 Oct. 2016. <https://www.ncbi.nlm.nih.gov/pmc/articles/PMC4837971/>

5: BASIC MENUS

Previous to the industrial revolution, few people ate three full meals daily. In pre-industrial cultures, adults generally spent the morning and/or early afternoon either in search of food (preagricultural tribes) or doing farm, home or kitchen chores (preparing the first meal from scratch). People didn't eat much if anything until *after* substantial morning physical activity.

The word "dinner" comes from the Old French *disner* which originally meant "breakfast," that is, the meal that comes after the extended daily fast. In English "dinner" has always referred to the *main meal* of the day, which in pre-industrial times always happened between late morning and midday. The word "lunch" originally meant "hunk of bread" and referred to an *after*noon *snack* – *not* a full meal – had between dinner and supper.

This means that in traditional cultures most people spent 16 to 20 hours daily in the fasted state and only 4 to 8 hours in the fed state whereas modern people spend more like 12 to 16 hours in the fed state, and only 8 to 12 hours in the fasted state.

Eating too often and fasting too little results in accumulations of excess nutriment and waste in the body, which promotes disease. There are many known benefits to having longer fasting periods on a daily basis, as well as periodic (e.g. 1-4 times monthly) 24-36 hour fasts, including:

- Reduced insulin levels
- Reversal of insulin resistance
- Increased rate of fat burning
- Stabilization of blood sugar levels

- Increased clearance of cellular metabolic wastes
- Increased rates of DNA and tissue repair
- Increased excretion of excess sodium
- Healing of the digestive tract
- Reduced systemic inflammation
- Improved immune function
- Improved healing of the nervous system
- Enhanced learning

We highly encourage adults to extend their fasting period every day to *at least* 12 hours, and preferably closer to 16 hours, and limit themselves to two main meals daily, all food eaten within an 6-8 hour "feeding window," generally morning and mid-day. For more information on the benefits of periodic fasting, look for my book INTERMITTENT FASTING.

> The superior human does not, even for the space of a single meal, act contrary to virtue.
>
> Confucius

Breakfast/Dinner

Regardless of when you take it, your first meal of the day breaks your fast. A break-fast generally should start with fluids or contain more water than other meals as this replenishes fluids and helps clear out sludge accumulated overnight and enlivens energy, like the spring rains.

We usually have medicinal tea, kukicha (twig tea), roasted barley tea, or some other herbal tea around 7 A.M. After this, we will do physical fitness training. After training we usually start our breakfast between 8 and 10 A.M., after a 15-17 hour overnight fast. Here are some breakfast ideas:

- Seasonally appropriate whole grain and bean congee (porridge, see Basic Recipes), containing beans, seeds, and vegetables or dried fruit.
- European style: Oatmeal or other porridge with fresh vegetables, nuts or seeds, or dried fruit and topped with fresh almond milk.
- European style: Oatmeal with beans and/or smoked fish, vegetables and/or fruits.
- Classic Japanese: Simple vegetable miso soup with soft-cooked rice.
- Whole grain pancakes or waffles with fresh or cooked fruit topping, and kukicha (twig tea) or roasted barley tea.
- North Chinese style: Steamed whole wheat buns or flat bread with steaming hot soy milk seasoned with miso or soy sauce and chopped scallions or fresh ginger.
- Scrambled tofu with optional plant-based sausage or smoked fish, vegetables and fruits.

Lunch or Supper

If possible for you, we recommend having your last meal finished at least 4 hours before you go to bed. Finishing your feeding cycle at least 4 hours before sleeping makes for better digestion, deeper sleep, and ease of awakening in the early morning, which is the best time for practicing meditation and breathing exercises (qi gong, pranayama).

For best digestion, finish your second and last meal by 6 P.M. – 4 P.M. is even better. Here are two formats I recommend:

- At least four to six different kinds of vegetables, cooked according to season; legumes, tofu, tempeh, natto, and/or fish or meat; brown rice or other whole grain, optional miso soup.
- Simple vegetable-miso soup or stir-fry with noodles (in the soup/broth) and/or 100% whole grain bread (try our steamed buns, or use tortillas, or loaf bread).

You can add wild-quality fish, poultry, or meat to the above as desired. For example, use a traditional fish stock for the soup. Here are some other ideas for supper:

- Italian: Whole grain pasta with tofu and/or plant-based sausage and lots of vegetables. If desired, toss in some fish, poultry, or game-based sausage (1-4 oz. per person).
- Italian: Polenta or millet loaf with roasted red pepper vegetable sauce and grilled tofu, plant-based meat, or fish.
- Sandwiches: Whole grain bread with grilled, baked, or smoked tofu, plant-based meat or fish (e.g. sardines or smoked salmon), and various roasted and/or naturally pickled vegetables.
- Squash-wiches: Try stuffing a tortilla or chapati with sweet winter squash (or sweet potato) and a light spread of nut or seed butter, as in our Vegan Sweet Potato Wrap on our YouTube Channel.
- European-style: Rye bread, kale and sauerkraut, and a stew containing roots, forest mushrooms, and one or more of the following: plant-based meat or sausage, smoked tofu or fish, or very lean game or pastured animal meat or sausage.
- French peasant style: Lentil and vegetable stew with, whole grain bread with olive tapenade topping, wilted salad. If desired, add plant-based sausage or smoked tofu or fish, or use animal-based stock for the stew.

- Greek Style: Greek lentil soup (perhaps using fish or poultry stock), whole wheat pita bread, and wilted vegetables prepared with olives and marinated feta-style tofu (without potatoes, tomatoes or eggplant).

Lunch/Snacks

- Fresh or dried fruits
- Roasted seeds or nuts
- Seaweed snacks
- Beans or bean products such as edamame, hummus, bean dips, roasted beans or peas
- Steamed or pickled vegetables (to accompany the whole grain or bean products)
- Whole grain sushi, rice cakes, bread, crackers, snack bars

6: BASIC RECIPES

> Food can never be too good and cooking can never be done too carefully.
>
> Confucius

Basic Whole Grain Bread Dough

Dry ingredients:
3 to 3 1/2 cups whole grain flour
2 teaspoons active dry yeast (more for a faster rise, less for a slower rise)

Wet ingredients:
1 1/3 cups warm filtered water
1 teaspoon unrefined sea salt (if coarse, dissolve in warm water)

1. Reserve 1/2 cup flour. Measure 2 1/2 cups flour into 12- to 18-inch stainless steel mixing bowl. Sprinkle with yeast, stir, and make a well in center.
2. Warm salted water over moderate (not high) heat until hot to the touch, no hotter than 100 to 110° F. Stir water to dissolve salt. Test with instant-read thermometer. If too hot, allow to cool.
3. Use a large spoon to mix warm water into flour' to form a soft dough. Add remaining 1/2 cup flour, a little at a time. When too stiff to stir with a spoon, begin kneading with one hand, using the other hand to add flour and turn bowl.
4. Knead dough in the bowl, adding as little flour as possible—only enough to keep the dough from being too

sticky or wet. Knead until dough is elastic, supple, and pulls away from the sides to form a smooth ball. Add more flour a tablespoon at a time, only if necessary.

5. Rest the ball of dough in oiled a 3-quart Pyrex bowl for a single batch or an 8- to 12-quart mixing bowl for a double batch. Cover a 3-quart bowl with a 9- to 10-inch dinner plate (oil the bottom to keep the dough from sticking as it rises). Cover a larger bowl with a larger upside down bowl. Or rest an oiled cooling rack over the bowl and cover with a clean, damp kitchen towel.

6. Let dough rise in a warm place for approximately 1 to 2 hours, or at room temperature for 2 to 4 hours, or until it has nearly doubled in bulk.

7. Gently punch dough down and knead a couple of turns in the bowl, folding the dough in on itself. If you're not ready to cook it, cover again, and let rise and double again. (You can do this several times if you like.) Alternatively, after punching down, cover and refrigerate up to 24 hours, then bring to room temperature and let rise one more time before proceeding.

8. Shape dough according to the Steamed Bun recipe that follows. Let rise one more time until it has doubled in bulk, about 1/2 to 2 hours, depending on ambient temperature. Don't let it over-rise. Cook according to directions.

Variations:

Slow-Rise Dough: Reduce active dry yeast to 1 teaspoon. Use room-temperature water. If salt is coarse or chunky, dissolve in warm water, then cool to 70 to 80° F. Let rise at room temperature until doubled in bulk, 4 to 6 hours in warm weather, 8 to 10 hours or overnight in cold weather. Punch down dough. If you're not ready to cook it yet, allow it to rise a second time, punch down, then shape and cook as directed for Steamed Buns or your favorite type of bread.

Steamed Buns

Unfilled buns can replace loaf bread, burger buns, English muffins, or dinner rolls. You can cook a single, double, or triple batch in 20 minutes using 1 pot and burner if you have enough steamers. Buns may be frozen.

You will need 2 stacking 12-inch steamer trays for a single batch, 4 for a double batch, and 6 for triple batch. Chinese bamboo steamer trays and large, stacking stainless steel steamers with tight fitting lids work well.

1 recipe Basic Bread Dough, from 3 to 3 1/2 cups of flour
Unrefined canola or other oil to oil plates or steamer

1. Oil two 9-inch heat-proof plates for a single batch.
2. For Standard or Slow-Rise Dough, let dough rise once in a covered bowl. Shape into a uniform 8-inch log. With a ruler and a sharp knife, cut into 8 equal pieces.
3. To shape, put 1 piece of dough in the palm of your left hand. Fold the top edge toward the center (as if closing the petals of a flower). Give the dough a quarter turn and pull an overlapping piece of dough toward the center. Repeat until smooth, round and all sides have been tucked in.
4. Place the ball seam-side down in your left hand. Cup your right hand over the top and gently roll to make a smooth ball. Seams should disappear quickly as you fold the dough in on itself.
5. Arrange 4 large balls of dough seam side down on each steamer, leaving 1-inch of space between each ball. Put each plate on a 10 1/2 to 12-inch bamboo steamer tray. Stack trays and cover.
6. Let dough rise in a warm place until doubled in bulk.
7. Heat 2-inches of water to boiling in a wok or steamer pot. Diameter of pot ,should match the diameter of the trays. If a

wok is used, bamboo trays should rest inside the rim but the water should not touch the bottom of the tray.

8. When boiling water is steaming, reduce heat to medium or medium-high, and start timing. Water must maintain a steaming boil for the entire cooking time: 15 minutes for a single batch, 20 minutes for a double or triple batch. Immediately turn off the heat. Let buns rest, covered, over the warm pot for 10 minutes to complete the cooking process.

9. Uncover. Remove buns with a spatula. Cool on rack or place in towel-lined bread basket. Store in sealed bags in the refrigerator. Use within 2 weeks or freeze.

10. To reheat, moisten and freshen leftover or dry buns, slice buns in half and wrap in an uncolored cotton-linen towel and steam over rapidly boiling water for 1 to 3 minutes, then serve.

Pressure-cooked Brown Rice

4 cups short- or medium-grain brown rice
5-6 cups filtered water
3/4 tsp. sea salt

Use a stainless steel or enamel-lined pressure cooker, never an aluminum cooker. Visit www.basicmacrobiotics.com for recommendations. Cover the rice with water and swish it around to wash. Drain off this rinse water. Cover with 5-6 cups of fresh filtered water (more in a dry climate, less in a moist climate). Soak for at least an hour, up to overnight. Add the salt. Cover properly and bring to full pressure over a medium high heat. Turn to low, place a flame tamer under cooker if on a gas stove, and cook for 45 minutes. Turn off heat and let pressure release naturally. Open lid and use a rice paddle to stir the rice top to bottom.

Boiled Brown Rice

4 cups short- or medium-grain brown rice
6-7 cups filtered water
3/4 tsp. sea salt

Use a stainless steel or enamel-lined pot, never an aluminum pot. Cover the rice with water and swish it around to wash. Drain off this rinse water. Cover with 6-7 cups of fresh filtered water (more in a dry climate, less in a moist climate). Soak for at least an hour, up to overnight. Add salt. Cover properly and bring to a full boil over a medium-high heat. Turn to low, place a flame tamer under cooker if on a gas stove, and cook for 50-60 minutes. Turn off heat and let the pot sit covered for 10 minutes. Open lid and use a rice paddle to stir the rice top to bottom.

Basic congee recipe

Serves 2-3, at most.

Place 150 g of brown rice, 100 g of another whole grain, 50 g of lentils or mung beans, and 25 g of seeds or nuts in a big pot, and add 6-8 cups (1.5-2 liters) of filtered water. Soak overnight. In the morning, bring to boil with lid ajar, then turn to medium for about 5-10 minutes. Add 1/2 tsp. sea salt, cover, turn low, and let cook for an hour or longer, until the grain is broken down into a more soupy finish.

If using a crock pot, cook on high for the first hour, then turn low and cook overnight.

Variations:

Grain and bean options: In addition to brown rice, our favorites include sweet brown rice (can sub for the regular brown rice), whole or steel cut oats, millet, barley, hato mugi (Coix lacryma), and cracked wheat. In place of or addition to the lentils or mung beans, add 1 cup of already cooked black, black soy, adzuki, or garbanzo beans.

For savory congee: Add any of the following: 1 stalk diced celery, 1-2 carrots, diced, a small piece of ginger, some diced leek or onion, chopped rutabaga, or cubed kabocha, buttercup or butternut squash. Let cook as above.

For a sweeter congee: Add some jujubes, goji berries, raisins, or chopped dates (if they grow locally). Optionally add a small piece of ginger or a cinnamon stick. Cook as above. You may top with non-dairy milk of choice, chopped seeds or nuts, or fresh seasonal berries or fruits.

How To Cook Tender Beans

There is no comparison between pressure cooked and pot cooked beans if you like them tender. A pressure cooker is a very worthwhile investment! We have listed recommended cookers at BasicMacrobiotics.com.

Pressure cooked beans:
2 cups beans of choice
filtered or spring water
3-4 inch piece of dried kombu/kelp to help tenderize and boost mineral content

Rinse and sort through beans. Remove any pebbles or debris. Soak overnight in water to cover by 2 inches.

Drain, then refill to cover by 2 inches. Bring to boil. Many beans produce a foam. Scoop that out with a spoon. Then add seaweed whole, or crumbled. If pressure cooking, close and seal lid. When up to pressure, reduce heat to a medium-low and cook for close to an hour. Newer pressure cookers can cook beans in much less time. We prefer really tender cooked beans for easier digestion.

Pot cooked beans: Use same method as above. Cooking time may be longer.

Seasoning: After cooking, season beans with sea salt, natural soy sauce, or miso.

Super Easy Tofu Recipes

According to Chinese medicine food classics, tofu fortifies the body's energy and blood, eliminates toxic heat (severe inflammation or infection), lubricates dryness, detoxifies, strengthens the intestines, and eliminates edema.

Many people feel at a loss with how to prepare tofu. Think of it as a soft somewhat bland plant meat that readily absorbs whatever flavors you add, just like a chicken or turkey breast, but without all of the bad stuff.

When you drain or press the tofu, it more easily absorbs the flavors of any added seasonings. To drain tofu, open the container, empty the liquid, and set tofu up on its side back in the container to drain more. To press tofu, use a tofu presser, or wrap the block in a clean dish towel and place it on a plate or board. Place another plate or board on top, and add a weight, such as a big pyrex measuring cup filled with water, a barbell plate, or a pot filled with water.

Simply Grilled or Pan-Fried Tofu

Cut tofu into 8 equal sized slabs by cutting in half lengthwise, than cutting each half in half, and each of those halves in half.

Season tofu with salt and pepper. Grill on a cast iron grill pan, or pan fry in little unrefined sesame oil for about 7 minutes, or until nicely golden brown, then flip and cook another 7 or so minutes.

Serve with veggies, or toss with a little good quality, naturally fermented soy sauce, tamari or shoyu at the end. Also good with a little chili garlic sauce.

Seasoned Pan-Fried, Grilled or Baked Tofu Alternative

1 Tbsp. garlic powder
1 Tbsp. onion powder
1 Tbsp. arrowroot powder, tapioca powder, flour, or cornstarch
A couple grinds of sea salt and cracked pepper, or a tiny pinch of optional cayenne
1-2 Tbsp. nutritional yeast

Combine seasonings on a plate or shallow bowl, and coat both sides of the 8 tofu slabs. Pan-fry in a little sesame or canola oil, grill on a cast iron grill pan, or place on a baking sheet covered with parchment paper, and bake for 30-35 minutes at 375 degrees.

Tofu can also easily be marinated in a baking dish with a natural barbecue sauce, or teriyaki sauce like Don's Teriyaki Tofu on our Basic Macrobiotics YouTube channel.

Simmered Tofu

This is a favorite tofu preparation, as we use the same pan to prepare all the veggies, and miso soup.

1 tub of tofu, drained on its side of excess liquid. This doesn't need to be pressed if you want to skip this step.
1/8 - 1/4 tsp. Chinese star anise seeds, or a couple pinches of ground star anise
2 Tbsp. naturally fermented soy sauce
1/2 inch piece of ginger, peeled, thinly sliced, then cut into little chopstick sized pieces
Small amount of crumbled sea weed, such as alaria, kelp, or bladderwrack

Veggies:

3 scallions, coarse chopped - use the whites and the greens
1-2 celery stalks, cut on the bias in nice long diagonal shapes
1-2 carrots, cut in half length-wise, then on the bias
4-6 shiitake mushrooms (or use crimini/baby portobellos)
Baby or regular bok choy or Chinese cabbage, cut thin on the bias

Cover a deep pan with about 2 inches of water. Bring to a boil. Add tofu, soy sauce, star anise, seaweed and ginger, and turn to medium. Let simmer for about 10 minutes with the lid slightly ajar to prevent boiling over.

Add celery, carrots, mushrooms and scallions. Let simmer another 10+ minutes until the veggies are soft. Veggies can be added with the tofu, but they will be much softer to eat.

Add bok choy or cabbage, cover, and let steam until just wilted. Remove tofu and veggies onto serving plater with a slotted spoon. Serve with brown rice. The broth can be enjoyed with added miso as a soup, or saved for using as a stock.

If you have fresh pressure cooked beans, the stock from cooking can be added to the water for a delicious broth.

Easy Quick Blanch / Quick Boiled (QB) Veggies & Greens

Choose a variety of veggies that complement each other, such as softer, juicier veggies with those that are more hard and compact. Below are some examples of vegetable and greens combinations:

- Bok choy (any variety) with daikon, celery, carrot, and shiitake mushrooms
- Bok choy (any variety) with broccoli, carrot, scallion, and red pepper
- Cabbage, carrot, celery, mushroom and onion
- Broccoli, carrot, daikon, and red pepper
- Darker greens like collards and kale with carrot, scallions, mushrooms, and cabbage
- Green beans, carrots, and turnips
- Carrots, beets, cabbage, and scallions

Fill a pot or deep pan with a few inches of water. Add a pinch of salt, and bring to a boil. Add cut up veggies, beginning with the lighter colored ones first. Bring back to a boil, then remove with a slotted spoon into a heat proof bowl. Rinse vegetables with cool water to stop cooking immediately.

Continue this process until all veggies are cooked.

Alternatively, if using a big enough pot, add veggies beginning with those that take the longest to cook first, such as carrots and celery. Then add mushrooms if using, scallions, cabbages, and finally bok choy. Cover, and let it steam cook for a few minutes, until veggies are brightly colored, but softened.

Thinly cut Chinese cabbage and red bell pepper can be added at the very end, or kept raw and tossed in the bowl of QB veggies. Dress with umeboshi vinegar if desired.

Once veggies are removed, the liquid can be used for a super easy, delicious miso soup that is great to eat prior to a meal as it helps stimulate the appetite.

Just add about 2-3 tsp. (about 1 tsp. per serving) of miso paste, such as a barley miso or mellow red miso. To incorporate the miso paste, place on a big spoon, and use the back of another big spoon to mash it into the broth, until it is all incorporated. That's it!

Add a little chili garlic sauce, or top with the shredded Chinese cabbage, or thin cut scallions as desired. Or garnish with thin cut pieces of nori seaweed.

Pressed Salad

The word "salad" comes from the Latin word for salt – sal – because in Roman antiquity a salad consisted of salted and/or pickled vegetables. Traditional Oriental medicine recommends little or no raw plant food, because it is harder to digest, but recommends vegetables that have been salted or pickled, if not cooked.

In fact properly pickled or cooked vegetables are more nutritious than raw because humans don't have enzymes for digesting cellulose, and pickling or cooking breaks down the cellulose in vegetable cell walls to release the enclosed nutrients for absorption.

5-6 cups cabbage (napa, green, or red), shredded
1 1/2 cups carrots, grated or cut in paper-thin matchsticks
1/2–1 cup red onion sliced thinly, or scallions in 1" pieces

1/4 cup celery, sliced thinly
1/4 cup radish (red or daikon), cut in thin matchsticks
1/2 cup cucumber, peeled, sliced into thin half rounds
1 tsp. sea salt *or* 1/2 tsp.salt + 1 Tbsp. umeboshi vinegar
1/4 tsp. grated fresh ginger (optional)
1/8 tsp. red pepper powder (optional)

Place all ingredients in a mixing bowl and gently knead with your hands to mix. Mound the salted vegetables in the center of a 3-4 quart bowl or ceramic crock. Place a plate upside down on top of the vegetables and set a large glass jar (1/2 to 1 gallon) filled with water on top of the plate to apply pressure. Press for 2 hours or more (longer in cold weather, shorter in hot weather). With your hands squeeze out liquid from the vegetables. Taste the vegetables; if too salty rinse under cold water and squeeze again. Serve 1/2-3/4 cup salad per person. No dressing required, but you may enjoy adding roasted pumpkin or sunflower seeds to the prepared salad.

Gomashio (Sesame Salt)

Ratio	Sesame Seeds	Salt
8:1	1 cup	2 Tbsp.
12:1	3/4 cup	1 Tbsp.
16:1	1 cup	1 Tbsp.

Suribachi (Japanese mortar and pestle)

Place sesame seeds in a strainer and rinse thoroughly with water. Heat a wok or skillet over a medium flame and add the salt; roast briefly until you detect a faint sweet odor. Place the salt in the suribachi, then put the sesame seeds in the wok or skillet. While the heat steams the water off the sesame seeds, grind the salt to a powder in the suribachi, while watching over and stirring the seeds occasionally. When the seeds are dry, stir them continuously and roast them until you can easily crush a single seed between your fingers. Add the seeds to the salt and grind them gently until they are powdery. Use small amounts as a table condiment.

More Recipes

Our YouTube Channel: Basic Macrobiotics

Our website: www.basicmacrobiotics.com

Our book BASIC MACROBIOTIC MENUS & RECIPES, forthcoming by mid-2016, includes many macrobiotic recipes.

Check the bibliography for other recommended cookbooks.

7: Harmonizing Yin and Yang

To secure the best health on a macrobiotic diet it is helpful to have some grasp of how to eat to support your constitution and balance your changing condition. Most basically, you want to know where your overall condition falls on the yin-yang (weak/cold-strong/hot) spectrum.

The following table will help you decide whether you have a basically more yang or more yin condition.

Feature	Yang	Yin
Complexion	More red	More pale
Thirst	Strong, desires cold beverages	Weak, desires hot beverages
Hunger	Strong, desires cold foods	Weak, prefers hot foods
Urine	Scanty, yellow, strong odor	Copious, clear or cloudy, little odor
Feces	Dry, hard, compact, infrequent, hard to pass, strong odor	Wet, loose, frequent, little odor, possible undigested food
Sleep	Sleeps on back or with little or no covers	Sleeps curled up or with covers
Energy	High	Low
Activity	Restless, forceful	Lethargic, weak
Speech	Loud, rapid speech	Quiet, slow speech

Feature	Yang	Yin
Mood and attitude	High spirits, assertive or aggressive, passionate, hot-tempered	Low spirits, passive, lacks motivation and passion, depressive
Climatic preference	Prefers cold weather, winter	Prefers hot weather, summer

Depending on your condition, you can alter your food intake in one or more of the following ways:

Food Group	More Yang Condition	More Yin Condition
Whole grains	Use more medium or long grain brown rice, pearl barley, corn, and wheat	Use more short grain brown rice, oats, and sweet brown rice
Legumes	Emphasize light-colored or larger beans, such as mung beans, green peas, and chickpeas	Emphasize dark-colored or compact beans such as lentils, black beans and adzuki beans
Vegetables	More leafy greens, less root vegetables	More root and ground vegetables, less leafy greens
Seeds	Larger and more oily seeds, such as sunflower seeds and pumpkin seeds	Smaller and drier seeds, such as sesame seeds and flax seeds

Food Group	More Yang Condition	More Yin Condition
Nuts	Larger and more oily nuts, more warm climate origin nuts, such as almonds, pecans and peanuts.	Smaller and drier nuts, more cold climate origin nuts, such as hickory, pine nuts, and hazelnuts
Fruits	Emphasize larger and juicier, warm season/climate fruits, such as various melons. Use more fresh fruits, less dried and cooked fruits, especially in warm or hot weather.	Emphasize smaller and drier fruits that have neutral or warm properties, such as apples, dates, raspberries, cranberries, grapes, figs, peaches, cherries. Use more dried or cooked fruits, especially in cooler seasons.
Animal products	Reduced animal meat intake; use moister or light-colored flesh from slower, lazier animals adapted to warmer climates; for example, flounder or perch.	Perhaps increased animal meat intake; use drier, darker, or more red flesh from faster, more vigorous animals adapted to colder climates; for example, salmon.
Cooking styles	Lower temperature, more water, less time; shorter pressing or fermentation	Higher temperature, less water, more time; longer pressing or fermentation

These are broad guidelines just to give an idea how you might adjust your diet to improve your overall condition, or how to adjust your food intake for different climates or the seasons (eat for the more yang condition in hot climates, eat for the more yin condition in cold climates).

Although useful for general adjustments and very simple imbalances, the yin-yang system has inherent limitations. A fully-trained Oriental medical professional will evaluate an individual's condition using Eight Principles: yin-yang, hot-cold, internal-external, and excess-deficiency. In addition, for complex conditions it is usually necessary to use at least one of the following further elaborations of yin-yang theory: qi, blood, and body fluid principles; internal organ principles; five transformation principles; and six pathogen principles (wind, damp, cold, heat, dryness, fire).

Once a proper diagnosis is made, specific treatment principles follow, and these specify the food and menu changes that have been found to correct the disorder through literally hundreds of years of experience. Each food has a thermal effect (cold, cool, neutral, warm, or hot), affects specific organs, and has specific properties, such as: nourishing fluids, blood or yin; supplementing qi or yang; invigorating blood circulation; resolving phlegm; clearing heat; or dispelling cold.

If you do make diet adjustments using the charts above, make them in small increments. For example, if you decide you may need more salt, add just a little bit more salt to your diet for a little while and observe the effects. Monitor the results and adjust again depending on the results.

Nothing in nature is static. Your condition will change over time depending on how you eat and live. If you start out too yang, and eat more yin, eventually you will become more balanced, but if you aren't alert, you may even become too yin. If you start out too yin, and eat more yang, eventually you will become more balanced, but if you aren't alert, you may even become too yang.

Don't be rigid and robotic about your diet. Stay alert and make changes when warranted. Macrobiotics is not a prison or fixed dogma, it is a practical, flexible set of principles for creating and maintaining health and happiness to support your prosperity, longevity and liberation.

> Plato, doubtless, reached his great age, because of his moral purity, temperance, and natural food diet:
> of herbs, berries, nuts, grains, and the wild plants of the mountains, which the earth, that best of mothers produces.
>
> Ovid
> Roman Poet

8: MACROBIOTIC FITNESS

For health, fitness and longevity, all ancient Greek physicians and philosophers recommended, in addition to temperance in food and sex, use of fresh pure air, bathing, friction of the body, and proper exercise. For the latter, Greeks developed a system of both intense and gentle activities that they called *gymnastics*, a word derived from *gymnazein* which means simply "to exercise or train." This word did not originally refer to what we now know as competitive gymnastics, but to any type of physical fitness training, which is why we still today call physical training halls *gymnasiums* or *gyms* for short. By the way, the word "calisthenics" appears to have been first coined in 1839 from the Greek *kallos* "beauty" and *sthenos* "strength," and originally referred to gymnastic exercises suitable for girls and meant to develop the figure and promote graceful movement.

Strength Training

Progressive resistance training (calisthenics, weight training) is a type of intense gymnastic and should be the foundation of every fitness program, because muscular strength is the foundation for all physical activity. If you only have time for one method of physical training, you should devote it to strength training, because strength training produces better overall fitness than either endurance or flexibility training.

Properly performed resistance training can significantly improve strength, cardiorespiratory fitness[1,2] and flexibility[3,4,5,6] whereas endurance training does not improve strength or flexibility (actually tends to reduce them), and flexibility training does not improve endurance or strength. Progressive strength training "produces greater strength, gait and balance improvements in elderly people than a flexibility exercise program."[7] Resistance exercise also improves self-esteem, mood, body image, and fatigue.[8]

In addition, strength training does more for health and longevity than endurance or flexibility. Muscular strength "has an independent role in the prevention of chronic diseases whereas muscular weakness is strongly related to functional limitations and physical disability."[9] Muscular strength reduces the risk of premature death from cancer and all causes in men,[10] and women.[11] Strength training is the only physical training method proven to retard and even reverse aging of muscles.[12] Hence, resistance training is paramount for macrobiotic practice.

Endurance Training

As already mentioned, properly performed strength training itself improves cardiorespiratory endurance. Sprint interval training is the most time-efficient way to produce cardiorespiratory fitness.[13] Sprint interval training involves not only less time but also less total body strain than conventional medium intensity endurance training. For example, a sprint interval training program would involve as little as 400 yards of sprinting once weekly. In contrast, a medium intensity endurance running program would involve jogging or running 1-5 miles weekly, which amounts to 4 to 20 times more stress and strain on for example the knee joints. Over a lifetime this means the medium intensity program involves far more wear and tear on body structures. Since a sprint interval training program puts less total stress on the body, yet produces equal or better results, it is more desirable from a macrobiotic point of view.

Mobility and Flexibility Training

Mobility and flexibility training exercises belong to what the Greeks called gentle motions. One should regularly use specific flexibility, mobility, and postural alignment training methods–hatha yoga (which derives some of its postures from European gymnastics [14]), systematic stretching–to enhance one's posture, self-image, strength, range of motion and freedom of action.

Deep Breathing Exercises

Many people breath very shallowly. Shallow breathing results in accumulation of waste carbonic acid in the blood, which has a negative effect on body functions. Daily practice of deep breathing exercises results in better pulmonary function and oxygenation and alkalization of blood and body tissues.

Although Greeks and Romans developed deep breathing exercises, studies of the breathing exercises of yoga, called pranayama, are most common.

Pranayama has been shown to increase handgrip strength,[15] lung function,[16] and cognitive functions.[17] Slow breathing (6 breaths/min) has also been shown to reduce blood pressure.[18]

Here is a simple deep breathing exercise:

1. Sit with a straight back.
2. Deliberately exhale and empty your lungs as much as possible.
3. Slowly inhale through your nose, filling first the belly then the lungs to full capacity.
4. Briefly hold the breath (1-2 seconds).

5. Slowly exhale through the nose with bated breath. Empty your lungs as fully as possible.
6. Repeat up to 10 times.

Martial Arts

Protection of life is a fundamental physical and spiritual discipline. Self-defense and martial arts training may save your life or that of a loved one in an emergency. Both men and women deserve to know how to protect themselves from aggression. Martial arts training is particularly necessary for men so they can fulfill their natural role as the primary protectors of life, liberty, women, children, elders, and property. In this era complete self-defense training must include training in hand-to-hand combat and the use of weapons, including firearms.

Martial arts training should focus on skills does not replace strength, endurance, or flexibility training.

Transportation and Recreational Activity

Whenever practical, choose walking or bicycling for transportation. For recreation choose activities that one can enjoy outdoors, such as walking, swimming, running, bicycling, hiking, dance, and various games. Spend time in majestic natural areas or woods as often as possible.

Cold Water Bathing

Bathing in cold water is a traditional health and fitness practice in Europe and North Asia. Hufeland recommended washing the whole body daily with cold water while strongly scrubbing the skin, and once weekly bathing in tepid water with soap.[19] Numerous studies indicate that regular controlled cold water exposure benefits immune function and anti-oxidant status.

Adding at least 30 seconds of cold showering at the end of a normal daily hot shower for 30 days produced a 29% reduction in sickness absences for participants in one study.[20] Ninety-one percent of participants in this study liked the results so much that they expressed an intention to continue the practice. Many participants reported an increase in perceived energy levels and compared the effects of the cold showers to ingestion of caffeine. The cold showers increase the body's release of metabolism-stimulating epinephrine.[21]

Subjects trained in meditation, deep breathing techniques, and cold water immersion for just 10 days had a reduction in blood levels of pro-inflammatory chemicals, and were more resistant to *E. coli* endotoxin.[22]

Subjects who took cold (14 °C) water baths for 1 hour thrice weekly for 6 weeks showed an activation of the immune system.[23]

Subjects given a 5 minute immersion in ice-cold water after exercise displayed lower blood levels of oxidized lipids.[24]

Another study found that people who engage in winter swimming have a 40% fewer annual upper respiratory tract infections than controls, and improved anti-oxidant status.[25]

Start your experiment with cold bathing by ending a daily hot shower with 30 seconds of cold shower. Do this for at least 30 days.

Once you get used to that, gradually reduce the duration of the hot shower and increase the duration of the cold shower, until you get to the point where you can take a straight cold shower for 3-5 minutes, during which time you should scrub your whole body head to toe with a rough wash cloth. Use soap only under the arms and in the private areas.

Get Grounded

Humans evolved in constant contact with the Earth, going barefoot or wearing natural fiber food wear, and sleeping directly on the ground. Modern footwear and lifestyles insulate us from direct physical connection to the vast supply of electrons on the Earth's surface. Scientific experiments indicate that our disconnection from the ground may contribute to poor health.

Studies have provided evidence that grounding – establishing a direct connection with the Earth – reduces pain, stress, cortisol levels, inflammation, blood coagulability, and urinary losses of vital minerals, and improves sleep, recovery from exercise and functions of the autonomic nervous system, heart, thyroid, and immune system.[26]

Shoes with plastic or rubber soles insulate us from the Earth's electron supply, whereas natural plant fibers and leather do not. Spend 30-40 minutes daily going barefoot or in natural fiber or leather-soled moccasins or shoes on the Earth.

Forest Bathing

Forest bathing means spending time immersed in a forest. Research has shown that spending substantial time in forests reduces stress hormone levels and blood pressure, and increases activity of natural killer cells that fight infections and cancer.[27] Spending 2 to 3 days in the forest provides health benefits that remain for at least 7 and up to 30 days after the forest bathing time. Get out into the countryside and forests as often as you can manage.

NOTES

[1] Artero EG, Lee D, Lavie CJ, et al. Effects of Muscular Strength on Cardiovascular Risk Factors and Prognosis. Journal of cardiopulmonary rehabilitation and prevention. 2012;32(6):351-358. doi:10.1097/HCR.0b013e3182642688.
<http://www.ncbi.nlm.nih.gov/pmc/articles/PMC3496010/>

[2] Steele J, Fisher J, McGuff D, et al. Resistance training to momentary muscular failure improves cardiovascular fitness in humans: A review of acute physiological responses and chronic physiological adaptations. J Ex Phys (online) 2012 June;15(3):53-80.

[3] Fatouros IG, Kambas A, Katrabasas I, et al. Resistance training and detraining effects on flexibility performance in the elderly are intensity-dependent. J Strength Cond Res 2006 Aug;20(3):634-42.

[4] Morton SK, Whitehead JR, Brinkert RH, et al. Resistance training vs. static stretching: effects on flexibility and strength. J Strength Cond Res 2011 Dec;25(12):3391-8.

[5] Santos E, Rhea MR, et al. Influence of moderately intense strength training on flexibility in sedentary young women. J Strength Cond Res. 2010 Nov;24(11):3144-9. PubMed PMID: 20940647.

[6] Monteiro WD, Simão R, Polito MD, et al.. Influence of strength training on adult women's flexibility. J Strength Cond Res. 2008 May;22(3):672-7. PubMed PMID: 18438255.

[7] Barrett C, Smerdely P. A comparison of community-based resistance exercise and flexibility exercise for seniors. Aus J Physiother 2002;48(3):215-19.

[8] Taspinar B, Asian UB, Agbuga B, et al. A comparison of the effects of hatha yoga and resistance exercise on mental health and well-being in sedentary adults: a pilot study. Complement Ther Med 2014 Jun;22(3):433-40.

[9] Volaklis KA, Halle M, Meisinger C. Muscular strength as a strong predictor of mortality: A narrative review. Eur J Intern Med 2015 June;26(5):303-10.

[10] Ruiz JR, Sui X, Lobelo F, et al. Association between muscular strength and mortality in men: prospective cohort study. BMJ: British Medical Journal. 2008;337(7661):92-95. doi:10.1136/bmj.a439.
<http://www.ncbi.nlm.nih.gov/pmc/articles/PMC2453303/>

[11] Rantanen T, Vopato S, Ferrucci L, et al. Handgrip strength and cause-specific and total mortality in older disabled women: Exploring the mechanism. J Am Geriatrics Soc 2003 April 29;51(5):636-41.

[12] Melov S, Tarnopolsky MA, Beckman K, et al.. Resistance Exercise Reverses Aging in Human Skeletal Muscle. PLOS 23 May 2007.
<http://journals.plos.org/plosone/article?id=10.1371/journal.pone.000046 5>

[13] Gillen JB, Martin BJ, MacInnis MJ, et al. Twelve Weeks of Sprint Interval Training Improves Indices of Cardiometabolic Health Similar to Traditional Endurance Training despite a Five-Fold Lower Exercise Volume and Time Commitment. PLoS ONE (2016);11(4): e0154075. doi:10.1371/journal.pone.0154075

[14] Cushman A, "Previously Untold Yoga History Sheds New Light," Yoga Journal 2007 Aug 28.
<http://www.yogajournal.com/article/philosophy/new-light-on-yoga/>

[15] Thangavel, Dinesh et al. "Effect of Slow and Fast Pranayama Training on Handgrip Strength and Endurance in Healthy Volunteers." *Journal of Clinical and Diagnostic Research: JCDR* 8.5 (2014): BC01–BC03. *PMC*. Web. 26 Oct. 2016.
<https://www.ncbi.nlm.nih.gov/pmc/articles/PMC4079989/>

[16] Dinesh, T et al. "Comparative Effect of 12 Weeks of Slow and Fast Pranayama Training on Pulmonary Function in Young, Healthy Volunteers: A Randomized Controlled Trial." *International Journal of Yoga* 8.1 (2015): 22–26. *PMC*. Web. 26 Oct. 2016.
<https://www.ncbi.nlm.nih.gov/pmc/articles/PMC4278131/>

[17] Sharma, Vivek Kumar et al. "Effect of Fast and Slow Pranayama Practice on Cognitive Functions In Healthy Volunteers." *Journal of Clinical and Diagnostic Research: JCDR* 8.1 (2014): 10–13. *PMC*. Web. 26 Oct. 2016.
<https://www.ncbi.nlm.nih.gov/pmc/articles/PMC3939514/>

[18] Joseph CN, Porta C, Casucci G, et al., "Slow Breathing Improves Arterial Baroreflex Sensitivity and Decreases Blood Pressure in Essential Hypertension," Hypertension 2005;46:714-18.
<http://hyper.ahajournals.org/content/46/4/714.long>

[19] Hufeland, op. cit., page 276.

[20] Buijze GA, Sierevelt IN, vader Heijden BCJM, et al., "The Effect of Cold Showering on Health and Work: A Randomized Controlled Trial," PLOS | One 2016 Sep 15.
<http://journals.plos.org/plosone/article?id=10.1371/journal.pone.0161749#pone.0161749>

[21] Kox M, van Eijk LT, Zwaag J, et al., "Voluntary activation of the sympathetic nervous system and attenuation of the innate immune response in humans," PNAS 2014 May 20; 111(20):7379-7384.

[22] Ibid.

[23] Jansky L, Pospisilova D, Honzova S, et al., "Immune system of cold-exposed and cold-adapted humans," European Journal of Applied Physiology and Occupational Physiology 1996 March;72(5):445-450.

[24] Sutkowy, Paweł et al. "Postexercise Impact of Ice-Cold Water Bath on the Oxidant-Antioxidant Balance in Healthy Men." *BioMed Research International* 2015 (2015): 706141. *PMC*. Web. 6 Oct. 2016.
<https://www.ncbi.nlm.nih.gov/pmc/articles/PMC4383303/>

[25] Siems WB, Brenke R, et al., "Improved antioxidative protection in winter swimmers," QJM 1999 April 1;193-198.
<http://qjmed.oxfordjournals.org/content/92/4/193.long>

[26] Chevalier G, Sinatra ST, Oschman JL, et al., "Earthing: Health Implications of Reconnecting the Human Body to the Earth's Surface Electrons," J Environ Pub Health 2012, Article ID 291541. <https://www.hindawi.com/journals/jeph/2012/291541/?viewType=Print&viewClass=Print>

[27] International Society of Nature and Forest Medicine, FAQ. <http://www.infom.org/faq/>

9: MACROBIOTIC LIFESTYLE

Nature is organized to facilitate the evolution of humankind and individuals to their highest potentials. As such Natural Law involves Natural Justice: those who discover and align with Natural Law thrive, and those who ignore or rebel against the Order invite disaster upon themselves and their lineages.

Since 1) humans depend on knowledge for survival, 2) the survival of knowledge depends on faithful transmission from generation to generation, and 3) we need morality to establish social order and pass knowledge to children, humankind is genetically programmed to develop degenerative diseases when we engage in behavior that undermines the social and sexual order necessary for raising healthy, strong, intelligent and capable children.[1] Simply, Nature delivers disease, degeneration, weakness, and infertility to those who engage in behavior harmful to children, family, and the life support systems of their habitats. Your ego may think this is harsh, but the Tao allows us free will to align with Reality or not. We choose our own fate. If we align with Reality rather than fantasies, we will achieve our divine potential.

Sexual Responsibility and Dignity

An individual organism must continually reproduce itself through growth and repair processes. Growth, development, health maintenance and life extension require continuous reproduction of molecules, cells, tissues, organs, and harmonious functions, over and over for the duration of one's life. When your body stops reproducing its molecules, cells, tissues, organs, and functions, you die. Thus, health and longevity are products of an ongoing process of reproduction.

To nurture and extend life, one must preserve, promote, support, and enhance one's reproductive ability. In Chinese medicine this is called nourishing life (Pinyin: *yang sheng*) and nourishing essence (*yang jing*). If one wantonly spends the precious reproductive essence (Pinyin: *jing*) in sexual activity and regeneration of sperm, semen, and other sexual fluids, one reduces the amount of this resource available for regeneration of other cells, tissues and organs. If someone lacking a surplus of this reproductive energy (jing) spends vitality in sexual activity and production of sexual fluids, he or she will deplete resources for growth, development, repair and reproduction of other body cells, tissues, and organs, and for other creative endeavors (arts, sciences, athletics, etc.).

Since the Life Force most powerfully manifests and propagates through our sexuality, we must revere our sexuality as sacred and divine. The biological purpose of sexual energy is regeneration – not degeneration – of oneself and one's kind. To lengthen life and achieve immortality in progeny, one must nurture and protect, not abuse and dissipate, sexual energy. Any behavior that produces or reflects sexual or social confusion, weakness, disease or disorder is correctly called *degenerate* because it causes physical, mental and social degeneration.

Under the influence of a harmful world view, many people have a very limited and heretical conception of sexuality. For humans full expression of sexuality includes all processes essential to healthy reproduction. This includes: maintaining harmonious relations between man and woman; intercourse; conception; pregnancy; parturition; proper breast-feeding of infants; and nurturing, protecting, and educating children for about 20 years until they become self-sufficient adults. Only people who have biological children and dedicate themselves to raising those children into healthy adults have the complete experience of sexuality.

Hold sacred, honor and respect your own natural biological sexuality as well as that of others. Science has shown that gender ideologies that creates confusion about this biological reality lead to mental and physical disorders.[2] An individual's sexual identity is permanently determined by the presence or absence of a Y chromosome and it is impossible to change anyone's biological sex with surgery or hormone injections.

If a youth spends their vitality in sexual activity, less will be available for manifesting his or her full physical potential. The European father of macrobiotics, Christoph Hufeland recommended continence until the age of 24 or 25 years as one of the effective ways to preserve the life force and prolong life. According to Hufeland:

> "There was a time when the German youth never thought of intimacy with the other sex till their twenty-fourth or twenty-fifth year; and yet nothing was then known of the pernicious consequences of this chastity, nor of many other imaginary evils of which people now dream; but these youths, increasing in strength as well as growth, became men who, by their size, excited the astonishment even of the Romans.
>
> "People now leave off at the period when these began. They imagine they can never soon enough throw off their chastity; and young persons, long before their bodies are completely finished, begin to waste the those powers which are destined for a higher use. The consequences are evident. These men become incomplete, half-formed beings; and at the period when our ancestors began to employ those powers, they, in them, are generally exhausted; they

feel nothing but dejection and misery in their weakness; and a stimulus of the utmost importance for seasoning life is to them for ever lost." [3]

Male and female genitalia represent complementary yang and yin poles of creative energy, like positive and negative poles of a magnet or battery. Heterosexual copulation connects the two poles, which generates energy for both partners, and can ignite new life. However, it is impossible to generate vital energy with two positive (yang) or two negative (yin) poles.

Avoid wasting the vital reproductive reserve in excessive sexual activity and ejaculation. After every expenditure of energy and substances (semen, fluids) in sexual activity, the body must invest reproductive (hormonal) resources in regeneration of that energy and those substances. If you expend your reproductive potency at a rate faster than the body can regenerate it, you will deplete that potency which is necessary for body rejuvenation. Masturbation wastes vitality without compensation or purpose, leading to depletion and degeneration.

Classical Chinese physicians discovered that promiscuous sexual behavior brings sexually transmitted diseases into existence.[4] Briefly, when a man and a woman have sexual intercourse for the first time the woman has a mild immune response to the man's foreign tissue in her vagina. With repeated exposure to the same man her immune system comes to recognize him as safe and does not react with inflammation. However, if she has intercourse with many men, she will have a series of different immune reactions to the invasions, and these reactions convert her urogenital system into a host environment that initiates, first, urogenital infections, later, sexually transmitted diseases, and finally, sexual organ cancers.

Biomedical research supports the Chinese medical view. For example, compared to women not infected with human papilloma virus (HPV), women infected with HPV typically have earlier onset of sexual activity, more frequent episodes of sexually transmitted disease and genital warts, more multiple sexual partnerships, a higher frequency of casual sexual encounters, and poorer sexual hygiene.[5] Of course women can also contract HPV from infected men.

Promiscuous and extramarital sex generally harms everyone involved, especially women and children. "Early initiation of sexual activity and higher numbers of non-marital sex partners are linked in turn to a wide variety of negative life outcomes, including increased rates of infection with sexually transmitted diseases, increased rates of out-of-wedlock pregnancy and birth, increased single parenthood, decreased marital stability, increased maternal and child poverty, increased abortion, increased depression, and decreased happiness."[6]

History and anthropology have shown that sexually promiscuous societies perish from disease and weakness, while sexually orderly societies such as traditional Europe flourish. Now that Europeans have embraced promiscuity, European civilization is perishing.

Before you set the stage for a biological wedding of sperm and egg, make sure that you have a righteous relationship with a spouse who loves Truth, understands the difference between Right and Wrong, and is committed to caring for the potential offspring.

Marriage and Family

Through marriage and care for children we can become *creators* of new life and agents of evolution and the self-realization of the Infinite Universe. Hence, sexual intercourse is rightly held as a sacred religious act, and reproduction must be handled with the greatest of reverence and care and only performed when we have confidence that the children produced will be physically and mentally healthy and robust.

Traditional marriage and family promote life and are noble and righteous. Never married men and women have substantially more disease, particularly heart disease, unhappiness, and shorter life expectancy than ever married men and women.[7,8]

Humans are naturally adapted to monogamy and harmed by polygamy. A comparison between monogamy and polygamy indicates that monogamy is socially superior, for several reasons.[9] First, it reduces male competition for women and the number of low-status unmarried men, which reduces rates of substance abuse, rape, murder, assault, kidnapping (of women), robbery, and fraud, sexual slavery, and prostitution. Second, it reduces the age gap between spouses, gender inequality, and fertility (a monogamous man can only father at most about one child per year), which increases the status of and resources available to women and children. Third, monogamy shifts male efforts from seeking wives to investing in children, motivating men to economic productivity and resource conservation (savings). Fourth, monogamy eliminates conflict between co-wives and limits childrens' exposure to unrelated adults, resulting in lower rates of child neglect, abuse, accidental death and homicide. Polygamy is harmful to men, women and children, hence it is heretical and unacceptable.

Before you have intercourse, consider whether you can provide the potential children with a healthy body and mind and proper support. If you have heritable diseases or disabilities, consider what you are passing on and how it will affect the children who will have to live with your choice.

Reality rewards those who create *healthy* new life with more life. Raising biological children within a stable marriage tends to increase one's life expectancy.[10, 11, 12] Having one's children at an early age (before age of 25) increases the potential lifespan of those children.[13, 14]

The sex drive represents the Life Force seeking greater expression in creation of new life forms: children. Only sexual union of man and woman can reproduce and extend life through biological marriage of sperm and egg. A child is the biological marriage of mother and father and is designed by Nature to require both the yin influence of mother and the yang influence of father for full healthy development to adulthood. Children raised by two loving biological parents maintaining a stable marriage run the lowest risk of physical, mental, or moral disorder, neglect, abuse or violence; are by far most likely to perform well in sports, social and academic development; and are healthier, happier, smarter, more capable, and more self-confident, as compared to any other caregiver arrangement.[15, 16, 17] Emotional problems are 4 times more likely for children raised by same-sex parents compared to children raised by joint biological parents.[18]

Respect for Ancestors

Each of us is a representation of our ancestors. We owe our very lives to our ancestors. We have scientific evidence that thinking about our ancestors improves our intellectual performance.[19] Set specific times, every day if possible, to establish a spiritual connection with your ancestors through dedications and prayers. It is beneficial to maintain an altar to your ancestors, recognizing that they live on in your very own life.

One should study one's family and ancestry, distinguish truth from falsehood (much of official history is false) and native from foreign elements, and actively work to preserve the biological heritage of one's ethnic nation, as well as the natural habitats that produced and nurtured that nation. One should also respect the unique ethnic national ancestry of others, and help them to preserve their own biological heritage and natural habitats so that their lineage can continue to thrive and contribute to human biodiversity. This includes non-human species as well. One should also consider Earth, Heavens, and indeed the entire Universe as ancestors.

Right Livelihood and Vocation

One should choose a righteous livelihood in accord with Natural Law moral principles and spiritual practices, i.e. non-aggression, truth, pro-life, pro-liberty, etc.. One should avoid or abandon any evil, destructive, predatory or parasitical livelihood.

The most noble occupations are those most necessary for sustaining human health and happiness, including: natural resource protection and preservation; farming and natural food production; home making and child care; cooking natural foods; crafting natural homes and furnishings; crafting natural fiber clothing; natural energy capture or generation; coaching fitness, self-defense, and martial arts; natural health care; and education aimed at preserving and expanding accumulated traditional knowledge, promoting healthy, righteous lifestyles, and improving people's judgement. Choosing farming as an occupation may increase one's chances of exceptional longevity.[20]

To discover your vocation (calling), you can start by asking your Self these questions, after meditation, on a daily basis: "What can I do to raise the quality of life for my people? What do my people need that I can provide?" Answers will appear in mind over time. Acting on that inner guidance is following your calling. If you persist in this practice you will eventually get a vision of your unique role in service to your people. Lawrence G. Boldt's book THE TAO OF ABUNDANCE contains useful principles and practices for discovery of your vocation and vision.

Music and Chanting

Positive music and chanting or singing can improve your health. Frequently listen to uplifting music and/or sing at least one song that inspires your gratitude, insight, creativity, generosity, kindness, virtue and alignment with Nature.

Meditation

In 1654, the eminent scientist and philosopher Blaise Pascal wrote: "All of humanity's miseries arise from an inability to sit quietly in a room alone." Research indicates that most people do not enjoy spending time "doing nothing" in meditation but prefer "doing something," even if that something is unpleasant or harmful.[21]

If you don't like to stop and meditate because your mind seems chaotic or unpleasant, this is a sign that you need to clean up your mind. Meditation gives us insight into our own minds, and how we must improve ourselves.

> Nothing, to my way of thinking, is a better proof of a well ordered mind than a man's ability to stop just where he is and pass some time in his own company.
>
> Seneca
> LETTERS FROM A STOIC

Every morning devote at least 5 minutes to focus your attention on the Present, detach from you thoughts and study your mind. Take a seat on a chair that enables you to sit with feet flat on the floor, back erect, and ears aligned with your shoulders. Key points of posture are:
1. Head lifted
2. Midriff lifted
3. Tailbone points downward or forward so that the pelvis forms a bowl containing the abdominal contents
4. Elbows are slightly bent
5. Palms on knees or hands lightly clasped in lap
6. Feet flat on floor

Let your eyes close about three quarters, and maintain a soft gaze on a point on the floor about 3 feet in front of you. Place the tip of your tongue on the roof of your mouth just behind your front teeth.

Bring your attention to your breath. Let the inhalation fill your lower abdomen, and with the exhalation let the abdomen empty. Mentally start counting your exhalations. Start with 1, 2, 3, etc. So you will inhale, then exhale and count 1, inhale, then exhale while counting 2, etc.. Once you reach 9, return to 1 and start over.

As you continue counting the exhalations, let all unnecessary tension drop from your head, face, arms, body, legs, etc. into the earth. If it helps you, think "1.....relaxing" (inhale) "2....relaxing" and so on.

Continue your focus on the exhalations, letting the mind do what it will without giving it attention, for about 5 minutes.

When you are ready to resume normal awareness, swish your tongue and saliva around your mouth and swallow, open your eyes, and gradually move your head, arms, and legs.

Just a short period of quietude like this can provide deep rest to your mind and body. Try it whenever you need a break.

Sleep

As with all other factors, both too little and too much sleep create imbalances in health. Sleep needs vary from person to person, but generally adults require only 5 to 8 hours of sleep per night, generally less in summer and more in winter. Young children and pregnant women may need 8 hours. Excess sleep leads to low energy, depression, trouble sleeping deeply or even insomnia.

For deep restful sleep, eat your supper at least 2 to 3 hours before going to bed, retire by 10 P.M., get daylight exposure at dawn, and make your sleeping quarters cool and dark (yin); even a small amount of bright light (yang), such as from a clock or nightlight, or too much heat (also yang) can keep you awake (yang).

Sleep requirements may decrease when you retire early, get early sun exposure, get adequate physical activity, and practice breathing exercises or quiet concentration meditation regularly.

Hufeland additionally recommended the following for sound sleep:[22]

1. Make the sleeping room cool, quiet and dark.
2. Keep the air pure in the sleeping room by keeping the window open during the day or use a air filter if necessary.
3. Lie horizontally in bed, with the head only slightly raised.
4. Leave aside all cares and burdens of the day when you go to bed.
5. Do not read or study in bed, as the ideas taken in before sleeping may disturb the spirit from rest.
6. Go to bed early, and rise early.

Hygiene

Use natural, non-toxic soaps and cleansers for personal hygiene. For reasons fully discussed in chapter 5, take a cool or cold bath daily, and a lukewarm bath once weekly. Scrub your skin with a rough wash-cloth during the bath.

Use cosmetics and cleaning products that are made from natural, non-toxic ingredients. Avoid chemically-perfumed products.

For dental care, floss daily and brush twice daily (after breakfast and your last meal) with water or a natural toothpaste.

Clothing

Avoid wearing non-breathing synthetic clothing directly on the skin. Wear cotton, linen, or other natural plant- fiber clothing for undergarments.

If climate and circumstances require it, use wool, leather, or other animal-derived clothing for outer garments or shoes.

Wear clothing that allows free movement of the limbs and does not restrict circulation.

It is best to avoid or minimize use of footwear having soles made of rubber or synthetic materials that insulate you from the Earth's electron supply. Whenever possible use footwear having natural fiber soles (e.g. hemp rope or leather) or another method for grounding.

Home and Workplace

- Choose a home built and furnished with natural rather than man-made materials when possible.
- Keep your home and workplace clean and orderly.
- Use natural non-toxic biodegradable cleaning products in your home
- Include some large green plants in the home to freshen and enrich the oxygen content of the air.
- Open windows daily to permit fresh air to circulate, even in cold weather.
- Keep your home orderly, especially the kitchen and dining area.
- As much as possible, strive to establish greater energy self-sufficiency and harmony with Nature by utilizing renewable resources and energy.
- When using a computer, protect yourself from potentially harmful electromagnetic fields with a screen-shield or other safety devices.

Arts and Crafts

Develop your aesthetic sense and skills with some art or craft, such as music, calligraphy, drawing, painting, sewing, cooking, wood working, flower arranging, and others.

Financial Freedom

Vivo parve: Simplify your life and possessions, but without extreme austerity. Seek athletic, artistic, moral and spiritual values rather than materialistic expansion.

Avoid debts and repay those already incurred as fast as possible. Live on a cash, savings, and investment basis.

Save money for support of self and family, as an affirmation of resourcefulness, self-reliance, and prosperity. Put some amount of your income, no matter how little at first, into savings to sustain yourself and family. It could be as little as 1% of your income, but aim for 10%.

NOTES

[1] Holbrook B, *The Stone Monkey: An Alternative, Chinese-Scientific, Reality* (Morrow Quill Paperbacks, 1981), p. 267.

[2] Cretella MA, Van Meter Q, McHugh P; *Gender Ideology Harms Children,* American College of Pediatricians 2016 Aug 17. <*http://www.acpeds.org/the-college-speaks/position-statements/gender-ideology-harms-children*>

[3] Hufeland CW, op. cit., p. 243.

[4] Holbrook B, *The Stone Monkey: An Alternative, Chinese-Scientific, Reality* (Morrow Quill Paperbacks, 1981), p. 263.

[5] Syrjanen K, Vayrynen M, Castren O, et al. Sexual behavior of women with human papillomavirus (HPV) lesions of the uterine cervix. *Br J Vener Dis* 1984;60:243-8.
<http://www.ncbi.nlm.nih.gov/pmc/articles/PMC1046319/pdf/brjvendis00004-0031.pdf>

[6] Rector RE, Johnson KA, Noyes LR, Martin S. The Harmful Effects of Early Sexual Activity And Multiple Sexual Partners Among Women: A Book of Charts. The Heritage Foundation, June 23, 2003. Page 1.
<http://cdn.freedomainradio.com/FDR_2899_Marriage_Partners_Study.pdf>

[7] BBC News. Marriage makes people live longer. Thursday, 10 August 2006. Accessed 16 October 2015 at
<http://news.bbc.co.uk/2/hi/health/4779267.stm>

[8] Lynch JJ. The Broken Heart: The Medical Consequences of Loneliness. Basic Books, 1979.

[9] Henrich J, Boyd R, Richerson PJ, "The puzzle of monogamous marriage," *Philosophical Transactions of the Royal Society B, Biological Sciences* 2012 March 5;367(1589):DOI: 10.1098/rstb.2011.0290
<http://rstb.royalsocietypublishing.org/content/367/1589/657>

[10] McArdle PF, Pollin TI, O'Connell JR, et al. Does having children extend life span? A genealogical study of parity and longevity in the Amish. J Gerontol A Biol Sci Med Sci. 2006 Feb;61(2):190-5. PubMed PMID: 16510865. <http://www.ncbi.nlm.nih.gov/pubmed/16510865>

[11] Sun F, Sebastiani P, Schupf N, et al. Extended maternal age at birth of last child and women's longevity in the Long Life Family Study. Menopause. 2015 Jan;22(1):26-31.
<http://www.ncbi.nlm.nih.gov/pubmed/24977462>

[12] Gavrilov LA, Gavrilova NS. Biodemography of Exceptional Longevity: Early-life and Mid-life predictors of Human Longevity. *Biodemography and Social Biology*. 2012;58(1):14-39. doi:10.1080/19485565.2012.666121.<http://www.ncbi.nlm.nih.gov/pmc/articles/PMC3354762/>

[13] Ibid., op. cit.

[14] Kemkes-Grottenthaler A, "Parental effects on offspring longevity--evidence from17th to 19th century reproductive histories," *Ann Hum Biol* 2004 Mar-Apr;31(2):139-58. PubMed PMID: 15204358. <http://www.ncbi.nlm.nih.gov/pubmed/15204358/>

[15] US Dept of Health and Human Services. Fourth National Incidence Study of Child Abuse and Neglect (NIS-4). Report to Congress. Section 5.3.1.
<http://www.acf.hhs.gov/sites/default/files/opre/nis4_report_congress_full_pdf_jan2010.pdf>

[16] Sprigg P, Daily T. Getting It Straight. Family Research Council, 2004. <http://downloads.frc.org/EF/EF08L45.pdf>

[17] Sullins DP, "Emotional Problems among Children with Same-Sex Parents: Difference by Definition," *British Journal of Education, Society and Behavioural Science* 2015;7(2):99-120.

[18] Ibid.

[19] Fischer P, Sauer A, Vogrincic C, "The ancestor effect: Thinking about our genetic origin enhances intellectual performance," *Eur J Soc Psych* 2010 Dec 1;41(1):11-16.

[20] Gavrilov LA, Gavrilova NS. Biodemography of Exceptional Longevity: Early-life and Mid-life predictors of Human Longevity. *Biodemography and Social Biology*. 2012;58(1):14-39. doi:10.1080/19485565.2012.666121.<http://www.ncbi.nlm.nih.gov/pmc/articles/PMC3354762/>

[21] Wilson TD, Reinhard DA, Westgate EC, et al., "Just think: The challenges of the disengaged mind," *Science* 2014 Jul 4;345(6192):75-77.

[22] Hufeland, op. cit., chapter 6.

BIBLIOGRAPHY

Aihara C. The Do of Cooking. George Ohsawa Macrobiotic Foundation, 1982.

Aihara H. Basic Macrobiotics. George Ohsawa Macrobiotic Foundation, 1998.

Benet S. The Abkhasians: The Long-Living People of the Caucasus. Holt, Rinehart and Winston, Inc., 1974

Boldt LG. The TAO of Abundance. Penguin/Arkana, 1999.

Campbell TC. The China Study. BenBella Books, 2004.

Campbell TC. Whole. BenBella Books, 2014.

Ferre J. Basic Macrobiotic Cooking. George Ohsawa Macrobiotic Foundation, 2007.

Flaws B. The Tao of Healthy Eating, 2nd Edition. Blue Poppy Press, 2008.

Fukuoka M. One Straw Revolution. Other India Press, 2001.

Holbrook B. The Stone Monkey: An Alternative, Chinese-Scientific, Reality. Morrow Quill Paperbacks, 1981.

Kushi M. The Book of Macrobiotics. Japan Publications, 1977.

Lao Tzu. Tao Te Ching. Feng G and English J, trans.. Vintage Books, 1989.

Lu H. Chinese Foods For Longevity: The Art of Long Life. Sterling Publishing Co Inc, 1980.

Matesz D. Powered by Plants: Natural Selection & Human Nutrition. Create Space Independent Publishing Platform & Integrity Press, 2013.

Matesz D. Intermittent Fasting: A Macrobiotic Approach. Create Space Independent Publishing Platform & Integrity Press, 2016.

Matesz T with Matesz D. The Macrobiotic Action Plan. Create Space Independent Publishing Platform & Integrity Press, 2016.

Matesz T with Matesz D. Basic Macrobiotic Menus & Recipes. Create Space Independent Publishing Platform & Integrity Press, 2016.

Minton-Matesz T. Make Every Bite Count. Create Space Independent Publishing Platform & Integrity Press, 2015.

Muramoto N. Healing Ourselves. Avon Books, 1977.

Ni D and Ni M. The Golden Message. Seven Star Communications, 1992.

Ni M. Tao of Nutrition. Seven Star Communications, 2012.

Ni M. The Yellow Emperor's Classic of Medicine. Shambhala, 1995.

Ohsawa G. Macrobiotics: An Invitation to Health and Happiness. George Ohsawa Macrobiotic Foundation, 1978.

Ohsawa G. Practical Guide to Far Eastern Macrobiotic Medicine. George Ohsawa Macrobiotic Foundation, 1986.

Ohsawa G. The Order of the Universe. George Ohsawa Macrobiotic Foundation, 1986.

Ohsawa G. The Unique Principle: The Philosophy of Macrobiotics. George Ohsawa Macrobiotic Foundation, 1973.

Puligandla R. An Encounter With Awareness. Theosophical Publishing House, 1981.

Puligandla R. Jñana Yoga: The Way of Knowledge. DK Printworld, 1997.

Rector RE, Johnson KA, Noyes LR, Martin S. The Harmful Effects of Early Sexual Activity And Multiple Sexual Partners Among Women: A Book of Charts. The Heritage Foundation, June 23, 2003.

Sprigg P, Daily T. Getting It Straight. Family Research Council, 2004.

> Tao is obscured when men understand only one pair of opposites, or concentrate only on a partial aspect of being. Then clear expression also becomes muddled by mere wordplay, affirming this one aspect and denying all the rest. The pivot of Tao passes through the center where all affirmations and denials converge. He who grasps the pivot is at the still-point from which all movements and oppositions can be seen in their right relationship... Abandoning all thought of imposing a limit or taking sides, he rests in direct intuition.
>
> Chuang Tzu
INNER CHAPTERS 2:3, Merton trans.

Printed in Great Britain
by Amazon